Being a Nurse

A personal guide from graduation to revalidation

LAUREN PHILPOTT

Registered Children's Nurse

Lantern

ISBN 9781908625533
First published in 2018 by Lantern Publishing Limited
Lantern Publishing Ltd, The Old Hayloft, Vantage Business Park, Bloxham Rd, Banbury
OX16 9UX, UK
www.lanternpublishing.com

British Library Cataloguing in Publication Data
A catalogue record for this book is available from the British Library

The authors and publisher have made every attempt to ensure the content of this book
is up to date and accurate. However, healthcare knowledge and information is changing
all the time so the reader is advised to double-check any information in this text on drug
usage, treatment procedures, the use of equipment, etc. to confirm that it complies with
the latest safety recommendations, standards of practice and legislation, as well as local
Trust policies and procedures. Students are advised to check with their tutor and/or mentor
before carrying out any of the procedures in this textbook.

**Use the free Learning Diary app from FourteenFish to record your notes and
reflection as you read this book.**

www.fourteenfish.com/app

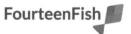

Typeset by Medlar Publishing Solutions Pvt Ltd, India
Cover design by AM Design
Cartoons by Fran
Printed in the UK by 4Edge Ltd
Last digit is the print number: 10 9 8 7 6 5 4 3 2 1
Distributed by NBN International, 10 Thornbury Rd, Plymouth, PL6 7PP, UK

CONTENTS

ME AND MY BOOK

Hi readers! Just wanted to say a few things before you start reading; I'll introduce myself and outline to you all the aims of my book and what you can expect as you read on.

My name is Lauren, and I qualified as a registered children's nurse in October 2014. I went straight into the job that I'm in now, although I did rotate to the Special Care Baby Unit (SCBU) for four months during that time. I'm now firmly back on the general children's ward, however, and despite occasional (sometimes frequent) wobbles, I really do love my job!

As well as this book, I've written several blog posts (mostly covering the things covered here) and also run a vlog. You can find this at https://graduationtorevalidationblog.wordpress.com/. Linked to this I also run a Twitter account **@grad2revalnurse**, so feel free to follow me or tweet about any similar experiences or feedback you might have – I'd love to connect with you!

But enough about me, I now want to tell you a little bit about this book:

When I first qualified I found it particularly difficult adjusting to life as a newly qualified nurse; I'd moved to somewhere that I'd never been, working on a ward that was very different to the one I'd trained on, and throughout my first three years I found some things quite hard to cope with. I realised that if I'd read a book that was a written on a personal level about some of the most common things you can expect when you start out as a newly qualified nurse, I might not have struggled as much – there is a great comfort in knowing that someone else has felt this way too. I could never find a book like that, so I decided I would write it. I believe that if I can help at least one other newly qualified nurse to know what they can expect along the way, and maybe make it that bit easier for them, then I'll have done a good job. That's what this book is all about; it's the book I wish I'd had.

Before we start, there are a few things that I want to highlight:

» We all know that our patients will always be our number one priority; everything we do is for them and I can't stress enough how much we all must strive to do our absolute best for our patients at all times. This book, however, is intended to help you, as a nurse, survive as a nurse. My hope is that it will help you on a personal level to cope with the aspect of nursing that will affect you, so if at any time you think I am neglecting the patients in this book or putting too much focus on the nursing team, please remember this: my aim is to help you, so that you can in turn help your patients.

» I can sometimes have a weird sense of humour, which will probably come across in this book, particularly in the parts that I found harder to write about. I figure that it takes a special sort of person to be a nurse, so I'm hoping you'll read it in the good humour that I am writing it in.

» I have included a lot of personal accounts throughout the book, as I find it useful to give a lot of examples (and so you don't have to listen to me bossing you around for the whole book!). During these I have referred to some patients and their situations, but I have done so in a way that they will remain confidential; I haven't ever included any names and have given away the bare minimum in terms of their conditions, but in some cases I've had to give more of a background. In these cases I have changed certain aspects so that they won't be identifiable; for example, I might have changed their age, gender or condition.

» I will apologise now if I come across as at all bossy or patronising – it isn't my aim, and sometimes I get very ranty if there is something I am passionate about.

Anyway, I'll stop wittering on now and let you get on with reading my book – I really hope it's helpful, and I hope you enjoy reading it as much as I've enjoyed writing it!

Lauren Philpott
May 2018

FIRST DAY NERVES

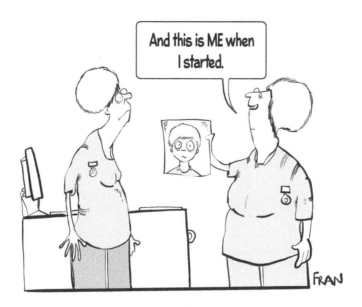

So you've completed your training and are about to set out into the big wide world of nursing. Firstly - congratulations! You survived your life as a student nurse, and you're only going to get better. As a newly qualified nurse you're probably feeling every single emotion all at once - relief, nerves, excitement, anticipation, absolute terror - I certainly did. It's a big step, but it's not as scary as you think it might be.

Nursing is such a rewarding job, which I'm sure you know as you've successfully completed your training. Whichever field you are in, you're about to commence a really wonderful vocation. You might have some tough times ahead, but if you can remain positive and remember why you're doing this, your career will thrive, and you with it.

This chapter will explore the important information you need to know as you set out in your wonderful new career. From your very first day, to your first experience of going it alone, there is so much to learn, and you're in for a really great experience. This chapter will also highlight the differences and similarities between being a student nurse and a qualified nurse, what you can do if you have a shaky start to your new career and the importance of always remaining positive. It will then end with a Q and A section which will address some of the most common concerns felt by student nurses when setting out in your new role. Enjoy!

Your first days

> 66 When I qualified I moved 180 miles away from my home and family, starting out somewhere completely brand new. I remember walking to work and not feeling nervous at all – something which I found very strange! I arrived early and was introduced to the night nurses, they took me to the staff room for handover and it just went from there. At the start I felt completely lost – all I could do was fight the urge to run home and cry. I was in a strange place I had never been, on a ward that I was not used to with policies that were nothing like where I had trained. It was overwhelming at times and a little bit daunting, but it wasn't as scary as I was worried it would be. There was a lot to get stuck in to and my colleagues were all so welcoming; by the end of the day it had become a positive experience. 99

Whether you're returning to a ward you worked on as a student nurse or starting somewhere new, one important thing to remember is that no one is expecting too much from you right now. The only thing you have to do at the very start is settle in and your employer will do their utmost to make this as smooth as possible for you.

Here are some handy hints to remember on your first day:

» Arrive early – you'll instantly make a good impression if you are punctual.

» Introduce yourself – this will provide a good first impression, and will help prevent you being called 'the new nurse'.

» Pay attention – there is a lot to take in, so pay attention. Don't worry if you don't remember everything, but if you focus on what you're shown, you're likely to remember a lot more.

» Take it all one step at a time – it can be very overwhelming so don't try and rush straight into things. Take everything at your own pace and just do what you can do.

» Stay positive – always believe in the power of positive thought. If you have an optimistic outlook things will be a lot brighter.

» Be proactive – in calmer moments (never say the word quiet!), check whether there are any cleaning or other day-to-day ward tasks that need to be completed, or simply spend time with your patients.

> 66 When I started working I kept a diary, and recently re-read it to remind myself how I was feeling during my first few days. At the end of my first day I'd written that I felt I hadn't done very much; however, the nurse in charge informed me that she didn't think she had either, and not to worry. Thinking back, I don't remember this being a particular problem and it pales into insignificance amongst everything else, but it obviously felt important enough for me to have made a note of it. 99

During your first few weeks you might be offered a supernumerary period (where you are not counted in the staffing numbers) to ensure you adjust to your working environment; this period will be extremely valuable to you, so ensure you make the most of it. You can use this time to find your way around, get to grips with the way your ward runs, familiarise yourself with the paperwork and the local policies and procedures. Before you know it you'll be managing your own patient workload and it will be like you've been working there forever.

If, however, you feel that you need longer to adjust, speak to your manager – please don't be worried, they are there to help you. Below is a handy list of Dos and Don'ts to help you in your first weeks on the ward:

Dos	Don'ts
• Take every opportunity to learn something new. • Ask about anything you don't know – there is no such thing as a stupid question and people will be glad you asked rather than going in blind. You must be comfortable with what you're doing. • Take time to focus on what you're doing.	• Don't sit back and let others do everything for you; you won't learn this way. • Never jump in and do something if you don't know how – this is risky as it can result in errors. • Don't rush around trying to do ten things at once; this will confuse you and you risk making an error.

Dos	Don'ts
• Get back on the horse – everyone makes mistakes, it's human nature. In times such as this it is very important to use the reflection skills that you learned as a student to understand why things happened and use this to improve your practice. • Ask for help if you need it; no one will think badly of you. If you need more time or support, speak to your manager.	• Don't dwell on an error – doing this will only set you back and put you off wanting to do it again. • Don't let yourself flounder; if you suffer in silence you'll scare yourself from ever wanting to try again.

66 The first week for me was all about learning where everything was, the way the ward works and meeting new people. I didn't have time to be worried as there was so much to do! I was not expected to take patients at the very beginning; I just had to settle in and get to know my new colleagues. Starting out can be very overwhelming but I don't know anyone who didn't feel welcomed into their new team (I know I certainly did). 99

Your first few days will probably be very busy sorting out the administration side of things (however, some employers like this all to be complete prior to starting your job). It might involve a meeting with HR to sort out your contract, your ID card and your uniform. Over the next few weeks you'll have IT training, be orientated to the ward and hospital. There will be a Trust induction, probably some manual handling training, infection prevention and control training, conflict resolution training; basically you'll do every study day under the sun, but you'll be so glad of this.

If you are returning to a ward you worked on as a student you will know your colleagues, where things are kept, how the ward runs, local policies and so on. Overall this can be very beneficial to you, but that doesn't make it feel any less intimidating. You might feel a little more protected; knowing the people you're working with can feel like a safety net, especially if you got on well with them as a student nurse. This can help to build your confidence and make the transition that little bit easier, but this does not come without its challenges:

» As a qualified nurse you might find that there is increased pressure from the start as your colleagues know how you worked as a student.

>> If your colleagues know that you work to a high standard it might be easy for them to forget that you're new and they might already have very high expectations of you.

>> You may not get as much supernumerary time and be thrown in the deep end a little more, which suits some people more than others.

If you are in this situation and you are struggling, it is very important that you talk things through with your manager. Don't worry if you are finding it difficult; it can be hard at the start and you need to do everything you can to ensure your experience is a positive one so that you can provide the best possible care for your patients.

Am I ready?

The step between student nurse and qualified nurse is a big one so it is perfectly natural to be worried, and it might take time to adjust. You might be surprised at just how quickly you adapt, but there is no shame in taking a little bit longer; confidence will come with time.

> 66 As a student nurse I remember a lecturer telling us that almost every student feels ready to qualify within the last six weeks of their final placement. I'm sure I felt this and in my final student days I was extremely sure that I felt ready; however, when beginning my first job I began to feel that maybe this wasn't the case. It felt like a step backwards because I was in a new place and had to learn everything all over again, but I picked it up quickly and once I had got into the swing of things it felt extremely natural. 99

At the very start there might be things that you can't do; for example, you may not yet have received your Nursing and Midwifery Council (NMC) PIN so you won't be able to give patients their medications. During this time you might feel a little bit dependent on the other nurses, but there are lots of other things you can offer to do instead to help your colleagues and care for the patients. For example, if your colleague is administering medication to your patient, you can in turn do a set of observations on their patient. This way, instead of feeling like a burden to your fellow nurses, you're being extremely helpful – it's all about teamwork! This will help strengthen your relationship with your colleagues, and it will do wonders for your self-confidence too.

Nursing is a very caring profession so don't worry that your colleagues will begrudge helping you – we all had to start somewhere! You'll be getting used to doing things that you weren't allowed to do as a student. This can be both exciting and scary, but don't shy away from them. Learning new skills is a key part of nursing and you should make the most of this period of development. People learn in a variety of ways; for example, some people like to jump in and 'do' straight away, whereas others prefer to talk it through and maybe watch before doing it themselves. Whatever your preferred learning style, remember – only do something if you feel ready.

Should I do it?

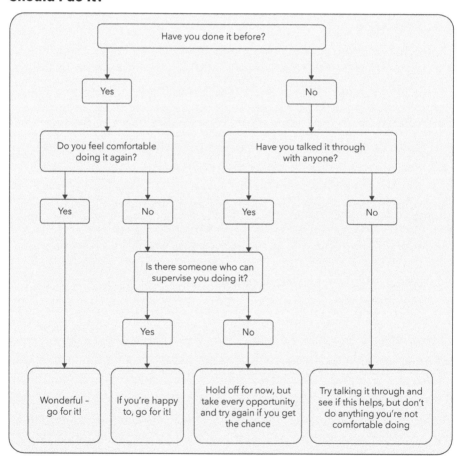

Although being thrown in the deep end can be really terrifying, with the right support it can have extremely positive results. Sometimes it takes being made to do a task to make you realise that you can do it, and it isn't as scary as you might think. Some days this might come when you don't want it, for example with a busy ward and short staffing, but other times you might feel like you are ready for a challenge. When appropriate, this is a great time to try – find someone who is happy to support you through it and give it a go. If there is a condition on the handover sheet that particularly scares you, ask if you can take that patient – it's a great way to learn and with the right support it can be an extremely positive experience. Below is a flow chart to help you decide if you're ready to try:

Going it alone

This aspect seems to be one of the scariest for newly qualified nurses – you might feel that you're suddenly left to fend for yourself. You go from being supervised by a mentor to being given a great deal of autonomy almost overnight, so you're bound to be worried. When you find yourself with your own patient workload you might feel an increased amount of pressure to ensure that you provide your patients with the best care possible. If this is you, please remember that although you haven't got a mentor to report to, there will always be other nurses on shift to support you through your day. You will never be 100% on your own.

The NMC recommends that newly qualified nurses be given a period of preceptorship which usually lasts between six months and a year. During this time you'll be allocated a 'preceptor' who will help you settle in and develop your skills and confidence – this will be expanded further in *Chapter Six*. This time of preceptorship, although officially lasting around six months, will in reality last around 2-3 years (in all honesty after three years I'm still not sure I've reached the end of my preceptorship period yet). You'll be constantly learning and developing, but it is the development in these first few months that will make the biggest impact on your confidence and ability to provide the best patient care.

> 66 *When I passed my driving test I remember my Grandad telling me that it is only when you're driving on your own that you really learn to drive. I feel like this same rule applies to nursing – it is only when you start to do it alone that you truly learn how. The foundation that you get from university is brilliant, but when you start to work you will consolidate all of your knowledge and learn how to be a great nurse.* 99

While some people are terrified at the thought of going it alone, others feel extremely liberated by the freedom. When you first qualify you might feel a great sense of empowerment because you're finally carrying your own workload without a mentor shadowing you. Maybe you find that as a student you struggled to work well under the pressure of being watched, so it is easy to understand why you might feel better when you're qualified. If that is you, that's wonderful – you're going to love your life as a qualified staff nurse.

If you are confident about your new role, that's great, but be careful not to become cocky. That will go down badly with your colleagues and you're more likely to make a mistake and risk patient safety. Remember that when you start you are a junior member of staff and that you must show respect for every other member of the multidisciplinary team. By respecting others you will earn their respect in return, and this will encourage a strong bond between you and your team. This will be expanded in the next chapter.

> **&&** *I still vividly remember the first time I was allowed to draw up medications on my own. I had spent two weeks completing the workbook my Trust had given me and had to do ten medications whilst being supervised by another qualified nurse, so I was eased in gently. That didn't stop me feeling the pressure though, and it suddenly dawned on me that this was it – I'm on my own here; it's my signature and my PIN. It was quite scary, but extremely liberating at the same time. It was a random adrenaline rush that I hadn't expected at that moment, and it was quite exciting! All of a sudden I felt like a real nurse.* **&&**

There are several differences between being a student nurse and being a qualified nurse, some of them bigger than others. These are highlighted in the table below.

Student nurse	Qualified nurse
• Working alongside a mentor, you have someone supervising you through everything • There are certain things you are not allowed to do, e.g. as a student I was not allowed to check BMs	• Working on your own, you have a lot more autonomy • Having freedom to do more can be exciting, but can be nerve-racking at the same time; once you've done something once though, you won't look back

Student nurse	Qualified nurse
• Being a 'student' can make you feel a little bit awkward at times • Doing shorter amounts of time on the ward, then being whisked back off to lectures	• Being able to feel part of the team – this is where you really make great friends • You're in a job that you're now doing day in, day out – you will get into the swing of things so much quicker and this is when you can really settle in

   My first contract was a rotation between a general Children's ward and Special Care Baby Unit (SCBU), and it was in SCBU that I noticed the biggest difference between being a student and a qualified nurse. On my placements in SCBU I was always working in the high dependency or intensive care rooms with my mentor, but as a newly qualified nurse I hadn't done the specific training in this so I was very rarely put in there. I loved doing it as a student, but not being able to when qualified was harder than I thought it would be; it felt like a step backwards. The team were always very supportive though, so if there was ever a time I wasn't doing anything I would go into the high dependency room and take the opportunity to learn about what was happening in there.

Whilst there are many differences between being a student nurse and a qualified nurse, there are also many similarities – more than you might have realised. If you find yourself worrying about the amount of changes, think back to all of the things you were doing as a student, and how many of them you are still doing now. See the table below for some of these similarities.

Student nurse	Qualified nurse
• At the end of your training you were taking your own patients (this applies to most placement settings) • You were always working alongside someone else, whether that was your mentor or a colleague	• As a qualified nurse, you continue to take your own patients • You will still be working alongside other nurses; your colleagues are there to help you

Student nurse	Qualified nurse
• You're always looking for something new to learn about • At the end of your final year you'll be working with students more junior to you, to share your knowledge and guidance with	• As a qualified nurse there will never be a shortage of knowledge or skills to expand • There always be students coming onto your ward, and they will be looking up to you as a newly qualified nurse, for reassurance

Qualifying can be worrying, but if you take it all one step at a time and remain focused, there should be no problem at all. You wouldn't have got to the end of your training if you weren't deemed competent, so you'll be absolutely fine as a newly qualified nurse. As long as you remember that your patients are your priority and know that you've provided them with the best care possible, you've done a great job.

A shaky start

Setting out as a brand new nurse is going to be stressful, so I won't try to tell you it isn't. Nursing is hard and work is busy, so not every day will be a good one. I'll explore this in more depth in *Chapter Five*, but I don't want this to be negative. I had an extremely shaky start to my career – something that I'd completely forgotten about until I re-read my diary. Almost everything I wrote regarding work at the beginning was negative, so I'm determined to make this book a positive one.

> 66 *Although my first few weeks were mainly positive, work very quickly got busy, I suddenly found myself struggling with a heavy workload and I ended almost every shift in tears. Unfortunately, sometimes this is the way nursing goes, but I was afraid to ask for help and was very hard on myself. This is why I would urge everyone to do what I did not do – ask for help!* 99

If, like me, you have a shaky start, please don't let this put you off. Nursing is such a rewarding career and you have to cherish these little moments of good; don't dwell on the bad. There will be times when you think 'why am I doing this?', and it is important to remind yourself why. Think of all the patients you've helped, the families whose lives you've made an impact on and remind yourself that you are a great nurse.

It is easy to get pulled down by work, especially if it's busy and with the usual poor staffing. You can very quickly get thrown into the deep end and this can go one of two ways. Either you can get stuck in and really thrive (if this is you, please tell me how you do it – I find this difficult even now!) or you can start to flounder. I really struggle in these situations so I completely understand why you are worried. There have been times when I've been thrown, or thrown myself into the deep end and it has had positive results, but that doesn't stop me from worrying the next time it happens. When it isn't a positive experience, however, it can make you take a massive step backwards.

> 66 *Upon re-reading my diary, I came across this account that I'd written when I'd been qualified for one month – I still remember this day as being one of the hardest in my career: 'I'm so unprepared for this! Every bed was full this morning so we knew the day was going to be busy. My patients weren't too bad and I was doing OK until around mid-day, then it went bonkers! I felt like I couldn't do anything right. My patient's mum was getting very abusive, saying that we were useless and that we were ignoring her child even though I'd spent so long with them. She was really laying into me and made me feel so incompetent, I couldn't wait for the shift to be over! I really don't know how I'm supposed to be feeling about it all.'* 99

Thankfully, that shift was a rare one, but something like that happening can really knock your confidence. The patient's mother (who is renowned for bullying the nurses) threatened to take me to the NMC and that scared the life out of me, even though I knew that I hadn't done anything wrong. I was reassured by my colleague that there was nothing more I could have done for the patient (she also explained this to the mother) and the child didn't ever come to harm, but that didn't stop that voice in my head telling me to just get out of the job there and then. I'm very glad I stayed with it, but it took a long time to recover from that shift. The next day I went out and bought a hamster though, so having a new little buddy helped!

Although you might feel terrified when you are in situations such as this, let me reassure you now that you will gain more confidence as time goes on, and it does get easier. As a nurse you're always learning, and you still will be even 30 years down the line.

On a positive note

Now you've officially started working you have lots of reason for celebration; you've graduated from university, you've secured a job and you're in for a wonderful and rewarding career. Although you might still be feeling nervous or worried about starting out, you need to take some time to feel immensely proud of yourself. You've worked hard to get where you are and you're going to be a really fantastic nurse. Here are some of the ways you can celebrate:

» You might have been used to being short of money as a student, so buy yourself a treat from your first month's pay. Whether this is a nice meal, a holiday or even simply some flowers, a little something special will help you to feel proud of what you've achieved.

» Have a night off - without essays or deadlines to worry about, you can now take one night to yourself and just do nothing.

» Go for a walk. The great outdoors has a lot to offer, which you might have missed recently through your studying or placement. Getting some fresh air and time to think is a wonderful way to reconnect with yourself before the reality of working hits.

» Spend time with your family or loved ones, wherever they may be. This will benefit both you and them; make memories, you'll be so glad you did.

» Reflection. This word is used a lot in nursing, and it is extremely helpful to do. Take some time to reflect on your training, write down your worries and think of ways to overcome them. Also, it's helpful to write down the things you enjoyed about your training, the reasons you wanted to become a nurse and the things you love about nursing. Keep it safe and dig it out when you need it.

Once you have finished your training, you can now start to enjoy life as a qualified nurse. You now have a 'proper job' (I use this term as this is how I now see my career - my previous jobs were simply weekend working while I was studying. I do not intend to disparage any other type of work in using this phrase) and can really settle down and enjoy your future. If you are a mature student you will probably feel very differently about this, as you might have had 'proper jobs' before now and for you, adjusting to working life is a thing of the past.

66 When I was a student I was talking to a newly qualified nurse who told me that she missed being in university. I, of course, thought that she was mad – who would miss the lectures, the exams and the essays?! However, when I started work I completely understood where she was coming from. I went straight from school to university, so I was so used to having set times off, I still find it strange that I haven't got a summer holiday to look forward to (unless I take annual leave, but I definitely won't be having six weeks), and adjusting to life as a proper grown-up was strange for me – sometimes it still is. Working shifts can be hard, but I find it particularly helpful to establish some sort of routine, even though this may be difficult. 99

When on placements you might have been working for only a few weeks at a time, with breaks for lectures or holidays. Now you can settle down properly. You might be a shift worker, or you might work set days, but either way you will now find it a lot easier to adjust to working life. Working shifts can mean that you might feel a little bit erratic at times, and adjusting from nights to days and vice versa can make you feel a little bit jet-lagged, but once you find your way of coping with this it becomes easier.

Common worries answered

Q: What if I forget everything I learned in my training?

A: This is a common worry, and it is very normal to be concerned about this. Once you're in the swing of working, everything will come flooding back to you, and you might surprise yourself with just how much you remember. It's important to keep in mind that no one expects you to know everything straight away; I work with nurses who have been qualified for 30 years and are still learning. Just take everything one step at a time and don't be afraid to ask for help. If you're not sure about something talk it through with your colleagues, they will understand exactly where you're coming from and it is better to ask than to assume.

Q: I'm worried about medicine management, what if I forget how to do it?

A: This is a legitimate worry for any nurse. Just remember your working out (for me it's $\frac{Need}{Have} \times$ solution or $\frac{N}{H} \times$ S) and you'll be fine. This is extremely important for children's nurses as the doses prescribed are based on age or weight, but for all types of nursing there will be medication doses to calculate. Get used to doing these calculations as a student and try not to feel pressured when qualified; you can always get your medications second checked if you are worried (this is policy in some Trusts anyway, and always is for intravenous medication). Also, always check the prescribed doses are correct using the BNF – doctors make mistakes too sometimes. Most importantly, just think logically about it; you'll know if your calculation is wrong – no 3-year-old will be having 30 ml of any medication. Don't be afraid to ask for help and take your time – rushing will not get you anywhere.

Q: What if I'm not good enough?

A: When you're starting out it is normal to feel like you aren't good enough; there are things you still can't do and this might be difficult for you. What you need to remember though is that you wouldn't have got to this point if you weren't good enough, so have confidence in what you can do. I know that's easier said than done, but just do as much as you can. One piece of advice that I always focus on is simply to **remember your fundamental nursing care** and you won't go far wrong. This advice came in a letter my grandmother sent to me when I was in my first year of university and this still remains the biggest influence to me in how I work. Below is an excerpt from this letter; the quality isn't the best, so I have also written it after.

Dear Lauren,

These are reminiscences of your Grandma (she has been thinking!!) over nearly 80 years, and experiencing of Nursing, Midwifery, Motherhood and Grandmother, and going through the phases of life. They may be of help to you in your years of Nursing.

I would love to give you many more hints and ideas on Nursing but it has all changed so much, but BASIC Nursing care does not change or should not.

If you think that this could be of use to anyone else, please feel free to pass it on.

Grandma

Dear Lauren,

These are reminiscence of your Grandma (she has been thinking!!) over nearly 80 years, and experiencing Nursing, Midwifery, Mother and Grandmother, and going through the phases of life. They may be of help to you in your years of nursing.

I would love to give you many more hints and ideas on nursing but it has all changed so much, but BASIC nursing care does not change or should not.

If you think that this could be of use to anyone else, please feel free to pass it on.

Grandma

Q: How do I know if a job is right for me?

A: Some people find that the setting they work in isn't right for them. Placements can go a long way in helping you discover where you love to work, but if you still don't know that's fine. When I first qualified I really wanted to work in SCBU, however when I qualified I found that I loved the children's ward and when I rotated to SCBU I realised that it wasn't for me. If that's also how you feel, that is fine; don't be afraid to try a few paths. However, and I can't stress this enough, don't let one bad day put you off an area of practice. If you've had a bad experience you might feel like you want to walk away and never come back, but don't dismiss a workplace setting because of this. Give it time; you'll soon learn whether it is right for you. If you really feel that you need to do something different don't be afraid to try – find your niche and you'll love your job.

Q: How can I manage my time properly?

A: This is something that I still sometimes struggle with, three years down the line. The key to this is prioritising correctly. This comes with time, but you need to use common sense here – your nursing instinct will tell you which of your patients is your priority and what needs to be done first. Take a step back and take time to think about what needs to be done and then do it in a logical order. With regards to time management, a lot of my colleagues use a time sheet; at the start of the shift they write out what patient needs what intervention every hour. Most people find that really helpful; however, I personally find that I write it out at the start of the shift and then never look at it. I do use it if I have a heavy workload;

otherwise just take time once an hour to ensure that you are up to date with what needs to be done. Just remember that you can only do what you can, and there is no shame in leaving the little jobs for the next shift if you can't get to them.

Q: What if it's too busy and I don't get the support I need?

A: The majority of healthcare settings are stretched with poor staffing across the board, so getting the support you need will sometimes be very difficult. You're part of a team though, so you're going to be supported by your colleagues no matter what, whether that support comes from the ward manager, your fellow nurses, the health care assistants (HCAs), doctors or even the ward clerk. This is the beauty of teamwork; there will be times where you are thrown in at the deep end, but you always have that team around you so don't be afraid to ask for help. During times where it is particularly busy you might find that the support will come following the shift or event, for example with reflection or a one-to-one meeting. Most importantly, if you don't feel supported make sure that you ask for help and don't do anything you aren't comfortable doing. No one will leave you struggling on purpose, so they might have not noticed that you're feeling the way you are.

TOP TIPS

★ Your first few months of working will be daunting, but you'll learn lots and adapt very well to your new role, and before you know it you'll be sailing along as though you've been there forever. Just remember to enjoy yourself and stay positive - everything else will fall into place.

★ If you're struggling, there is absolutely nothing wrong with asking for help; speak to your manager or senior nurse about what you're having difficulty with and they can then work with you to explore your options. It's far better to speak up early than to flounder, both for yourself and for your patients.

★ If you don't feel ready to do something, you don't have to do it - just ask one of your colleagues who will be happy to help. Don't shy away from it forever, though, because sometimes being thrown in at the deep end is the best way to learn.

★ Whether you're starting somewhere new or returning to a placement, remember that no one is expecting too much of you on day one. Give yourself time to find your feet and settle into your new role; putting lots of pressure on yourself will only add to your stress. You'll get there in your own time, don't worry!

★ When you're a junior member of staff you'll have lots of experienced staff to look up to, but soon there will be newer, even more junior members of staff joining. These nurses will then be looking up to you, so remember how you felt in their position and help them in the same way you were helped. This way you'll make great friends and enable everyone to have a positive experience.

TEAMWORK

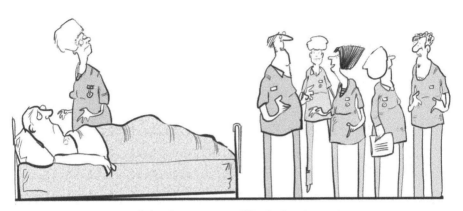

Doing things by yourself for the first time

Nursing is a career in which you're almost always going to be working within a team of people, whether this is other nurses, doctors or members of a multidisciplinary team. This chapter will highlight why teamwork is important for both yourself and for your patients; it will explore your nursing team and other teams you are likely to be working alongside, how you can support each other and how you can ensure your relationships are positive ones.

Working as part of a strong and supportive team is so important in ensuring that you are able to provide your patients with the best possible care, so with this in mind I will also explore ways that you can help build a stronger team, how to effectively communicate with the members of other teams you're likely to work alongside and the importance of working together to ensure patients are cared for in the best possible way.

The importance of teamwork

> 66 *A few months before I moved, I planned a day to explore my soon-to-be new home and visit my new ward. I had never been to the area before and I didn't know anyone I would be working with so was very apprehensive about starting out. I was shown around by a band 6 nurse who was extremely kind and*

welcoming and I remember driving home, knowing that I had made the right decision. A few months later, on the weekend before I was due to start, I went to visit the ward once more to find out my shifts. I then met another band 6 nurse who was also extremely kind and later that day I received a message from her saying that I was welcome to visit the ward over the weekend for a cup of tea and to meet my new colleagues. Little gestures like this meant the world at that time and I instantly knew that my new team were going to be wonderful. 🙿

Nurses are caring in our very nature, so be assured that you're going to be welcomed into your new team with open arms. Whatever setting you work in you will always have a team around you; your colleagues will help support and guide you, and you, them. Below are four reasons why being part of a team is vital, and wonderful:

Time-keeping can be difficult if things don't go to plan, but if you get tied up with something in particular, your colleagues will be on hand to help with any patient care that needs to be fulfilled. Likewise, you can return the favour when required – this goes a long way in forming a strong team.

Emotionally, nursing can be tough at times. As colleagues you will help each other through difficult situations and you will celebrate the good times together. For me, this is one of the most rewarding aspects of being part of a team – it's an amazing feeling!

As part of a supportive team you will soon find that your self-esteem and confidence have improved; this will ensure that every aspect of nursing will remain positive for both yourself and your patients.

More time is spent with your colleagues than with anyone else, so forming a strong bond with them will help ensure that you are all able to remain happy, work effectively and provide the best patient care possible.

🙿 *I've never worked anywhere (as a qualified nurse or as a student) where the team haven't been extremely welcoming. The people I work with now are really amazing and I fitted in straight away; they made the transition so easy for me. There are times when work is hard, but our team is brilliant and no matter what the situation, we can always get each other through it.* 🙿

Working as part of a team allows for a great deal of support for those who need it; whether this is a colleague, yourself or a patient. When you are working alongside caring and supportive people it becomes so much easier to share a burden or even your workload when required. In *Chapter Seven* I will be exploring 'burnout' and how it can affect you or your colleagues. In times such as this it is extremely important to be surrounded by a supportive team; people who you can rely on to help you through a difficult time. Equally, if you know of a colleague who is struggling, being there for them as a source of support and friendship will go a long way, and your team will become closer because of it.

When you have a good team around you, you know you're going to have a great shift no matter what is going on because you will all pull together. Nurses help each other, not because we have to but because we want to. If we share the workload when times get tough it becomes remarkably easier to manage and the friendships grow stronger. My favourite aspect of working within a team comes in these little moments where things don't seem positive; one small gesture, whether it be help with patient care, or even a smile or hug from a colleague can make everything so much better, and can remind you that you do an amazing job and have wonderful colleagues.

> **❝** *There have been times where work has been incredibly busy and I feel like I don't know if I'm coming or going. My department has two parts - the main ward and the assessment unit. Both are separate entities but are joined to each other and the same staff members work on both. During one memorable shift I was on the assessment unit on my own and suddenly found myself with a heavy workload that I was struggling to stay on top of. I went to speak to the nurse in charge as I was concerned about the safety of the patients, and before I knew it I had three colleagues offering to help with the patient care so that I could take some time to get on top of everything else. This was so gratefully appreciated and really instilled in me the knowledge that my colleagues are wonderful and always willing to help each other. Teamwork is so vital not only in helping each other through a busy day, but also in maintaining patient safety, and that's the most important reason we do it. **❞***

One of the most rewarding aspects for me of working within a team is the relationships you build with your colleagues and how they affect not only your practice but you as a person. I am constantly amazed by my colleagues and the wonderful work they do; they are so knowledgeable and always willing to share this with others. Their practice has a massive influence on the way I work, making me constantly strive to become a better nurse.

The nursing team

The colleagues you work alongside mainly will usually be your fellow nursing team (including both qualified nurses and healthcare assistants), and these people will teach you the most as you progress in your career. It's natural that you will form closer bonds with certain people - that's human nature, but it is important to remember that everyone you work alongside has something valuable that they contribute towards the team.

Here are some of the different 'types' of nurses you might recognise - of course, these are stereotypes and you'll be able to make your own judgements about the people you'll meet along the way, but everyone is unique and all make a wonderful contribution to your nursing team:

The Experienced Nurse	This nurse has lots of experience under their belt, and they are always willing to share this with anyone. They may have been qualified for many years, or they might not have been qualified for as long as you think, but they've learned a lot of little tricks in their time and their wisdom is passed down to everyone who needs it. They can be a little bit stuck in their ways at times, but you know that their number one priority will always be the patient, followed closely by their colleagues.
The Nervous Nurse	This nurse might be brand new, or they might have been qualified for a little while but are still not the most confident. They will have a permanent look of fear in their eyes and worry about everything, but will always do their utmost for every patient. These nurses don't stick around for too long before they slowly start to evolve into another type of nurse (and they can just as quickly come back), but they will never forget that time when they were new to this wonderful world of nursing.

The Wonder Nurse	There is always at least one 'wonder nurse' in every department (although every nurse is wonderful of course!). This nurse is the one who everyone looks up to; they are an endless source of knowledge and advice and can always be relied upon. The patient care they provide is always amazing and everyone, from patients to staff, loves them. Their handy hints will stay with you for your whole career, and if you become even half the nurse they are, you'll be extremely proud of what you've achieved.
The "I'll Just Do This One More Thing" Nurse	Every ward has at least one of these nurses. They will very rarely be spotted at the nurses' station as they are always busy doing something or other. It might take them that little bit longer to perform a task and time management might not be their strong suit, but they will always have the patient's best interests at the forefront of their minds. They have a heart of gold and will do absolutely anything for anyone.
The Determined Nurse	This nurse is usually seen running around the ward like they're on a mission and they are intent on completing every task they set themselves. Delegation isn't something they are well-known for and they are very good at performing tasks efficiently. Everything they do is to make their patient's stay a positive experience and they will always go above and beyond, even if this means they miss out on their breaks or finish late.
The Chilled-out Nurse	This nurse is not fazed by anything and always has a smile on their face, no matter how busy they are. They've probably been working for a while and don't worry about the little things that they can't change. They will always do what they can for their patients and colleagues, but are aware of their limits and aren't afraid to delegate when appropriate. They will always give their patients the best care they possibly can and everything is done exactly when they need it.

It is this wonderful mix of people that makes a really great team; every nurse has something unique that they can contribute to ensure the patients receive the best care they possibly can. It also allows people to work well together and inspire each other; the 'Nervous Nurse' will look up to the 'Experienced Nurse' who in turn will enjoy sharing their wisdom, the 'Determined Nurse' will be able to help the '"I'll Just Do This One More Thing" Nurse' when they have lots to do and the 'Chilled-out Nurse' will remain calm regardless of how busy it is, which in turn will help everyone else to keep composure.

66 *One of my most memorable shifts happened around a year after I qualified; we came on shift to very poor staffing and a full ward. We each had six patients and we knew it would be a busy day – we didn't stop! But we had a really amazing team: myself ('the New Nurse'), two 'wonder nurses' and a fantastic health care assistant. Our nurse in charge was the most chilled-out nurse I've ever worked with, and despite the heavy workload it was impossible to become stressed. We worked amazingly well as a team, being able not just to provide basic care for our patients but to go the extra mile, and we even managed to fit in time for tea and biscuits before the shift ended. It is this kind of teamwork that makes for an extremely rewarding shift and it's this teamwork that means the most. I'll always regard this as one of my favourite shifts for that very reason – we are an amazing team!* 99

Finding your role within the team

When you're new to a department, it might take you a little bit of time to find your feet (as explored in *Chapter One*) and establish your role within the team. In my opinion, if you have a good work ethic and are a 'team player', you're already over half way there.

There is some aspect of hierarchy within the nursing team, but that's not to say that those who are a higher 'band' are any more important than those of a lower one. Although the roles for each band can be very different, this mixture is required in order for the working environment to run smoothly. Having a mixture of skills is important both for patient safety and staff development and allows nurses of different levels of experience to work together efficiently; the junior members of staff can learn a lot from those who have more experience and can then in turn pass that on to others when appropriate.

No matter how junior you are, there will always be something that you can contribute to the team. You might have learned a skill during your training that some nurses might be unfamiliar with, or your knowledge on a certain illness or condition might be more in-depth than that of one of your colleagues. Offering to help and taking these opportunities is an extremely important way of ensuring your role within the team is a positive one.

> 66 *You might remember me saying in* Chapter One *that my first job was on a rotational post to a general children's ward and SCBU. Not long after I had returned to the general children's ward myself and the nurse in charge were stood at the desk when a doctor asked my colleague if she wouldn't mind doing a blood gas on a baby - something that is performed very frequently in SCBU. The nurse in charge pointed out that although she is a senior nurse, I might be better at doing this because of my recent rotation. This meant a lot to me because that nurse is one of the best I've ever worked with, and the fact that she had acknowledged a skill of mine really helped me to feel like an important part of the team.* 99

Below are some of the ways that you can help provide a positive contribution to your team:

» Share your knowledge - as mentioned above, there are many things you might have learned during your training that your new colleagues don't know about, so don't be afraid to pass on your hints and tips.

» Offer to help - this was touched upon in the previous chapter, but I'll reiterate it here; offer to help your colleagues, especially if they are doing something for you, e.g IV medications before you're signed off. Helping with something as simple as observations is a great way to ensure you become a positive contribution to your team.

» Be a team player - even though patients are allocated their own nurse, that doesn't mean you don't have to help them. If someone presses their call bell and their nurse is busy, assist the patient. Don't make them wait for their nurse if you are free and able to help. This might seem simple enough, but sometimes we (and our patients) can become too fixated on which nurse is caring for which patient and teamwork can go out the window. If you're unsure of the plan of care, check with the patient's named nurse, but there is no reason you can't assist. Sorry for the rant on this one, but it's a real pet peeve of mine.

» Be friendly - this one's simple enough; if you are polite and approachable you'll instantly provide positivity and support to your colleagues, and you'll be able to form great friendships because of it.

Lone working

Being part of a supportive team is highly important if you are a lone worker. Whether this is in the community or on a ward, there will be times when you have to work alone. In the community these situations will be frequent, whereas in a ward setting they will be more fleeting. Whether you work alone often or not, it is extremely important that you have a team around you to ensure your safety. If you are a community worker you should always tell your colleagues where you are going, at what time, and when they should expect you back. Likewise, if your colleague has been out for a long time you should always check on them to ensure they are safe. If you have any concerns, you should escalate these in the appropriate ways (these will be specific to each Trust, so find out your local policies). This also goes for if you are working on a ward – if you're going in to see a patient who is known to be volatile, always tell a colleague where you are going, and if necessary go in two at a time.

> ❝ On our ward, particularly on night shifts, we will always ensure that we tell someone what room we are going to – especially if we know the patient or their parents have been argumentative or rude. There have been times where we have been told to always go two at a time to certain patients, and have a system whereby if the nurse hasn't returned within five minutes we will go to the room to ensure they are OK, and if needed we will find a reason to pull them out, for example asking if they have the drug cupboard keys or to check a medication. This way we can ensure each other's safety. ❞

The multidisciplinary team

As well as your fellow nurses, there are many other members of the multidisciplinary team (MDT) you will work alongside. This includes doctors, dietitians, physiotherapists, pharmacists, ward clerks, receptionists, porters and domestic workers, amongst others. The amount you work with each of these colleagues will vary, but in order for everything to run smoothly it is very important to maintain a good relationship with everyone you work with. Respect goes a long way when working with different people, and it is integral to remember that everyone has an important role to play.

Secondary to our nursing colleagues, we work very closely alongside the doctors. When the relationship between the nursing and medical team is a positive one you will find that things run much more smoothly and the morale on the ward is a lot more positive. You will also find great opportunities to learn from the doctors and that they are more willing to teach you about conditions and illnesses if your relationship is good. By building a good rapport with them, doctors are more likely to trust your opinion and take on board your advice. Doctors who believe nurses to be beneath them are very dated and thankfully rare, but you can help eradicate this attitude quickly by offering your help and showing respect. Of course this is a two-way street, but in general if you respect the doctors, they will respect you, and most are very grateful for your help and advice – even if they don't always show it.

> 66 When we build a good relationship with our doctors it becomes so much easier to work alongside each other; they are grateful for our help and advice and in return they are happy to share with us their knowledge. In an earlier personal account I wrote about a busy shift on the assessment unit. During this shift I was working with a senior house officer (SHO) who I didn't know very well at the time; I now know her to be a fantastic doctor, a great source of support and a good friend. She could tell that I was struggling with the heavy workload so she took me aside, gave me a hug and offered to help with nursing care. I've never known a doctor to do this before so was quite taken aback, but to me this highlighted more than anything else that if doctors and nurses work together, the optimum patient care will be achieved and a positive work environment will be created. 99

Working alongside doctors can sometimes be difficult, as their training teaches them to look at things in a different way, but overall working with each other allows everything to run much more smoothly. When there is a mutual understanding from both sides, a clear plan can be made involving the medical team, the nursing team and of course, the patient/family team. There are some instances where doctors and nurses are required to work together, for example when giving treatments or breaking bad news, and it is during these times, the latter in particular, that it is extremely important that the relationship is good; we are there to support each other. This will be explored fully in *Chapter Four*.

As well as doctors, there are also several other teams that we as nurses work alongside. The teams you work closely with will differ depending on which department you work in, so I won't delve too deeply into these – that would get very long and boring. Instead I will briefly explore the roles of some of the most common specialities and highlight the importance of developing good relationships with them:

» **Ward clerks** - most wards have ward clerks, and these people are fantastic; without them we would have so much extra paperwork to do (and when would we fit in patient care?!). They do so much for us, from answering the phone to ordering supplies, even running errands if we simply do not have time, and it can be easy to forget how important their work is in allowing us to do our jobs effectively.

» **Pharmacists** - if you have any patient requiring medication, then you will encounter a pharmacist along the way. I am in complete awe of pharmacy staff - they can reel off a long list of medications and even side-effects at the drop of a hat. They are extremely knowledgeable, are responsible for ensuring that the patients are topped up with all of their medications, and are hot on ensuring the doses are correct. Not only this, but they are a great source of help if there are any weird and wonderful medications that you need to try to get hold of - something that always seems to happen out of hours!

» **Dietitians** - not every department will work alongside dietitians, but if you do you will know what an amazing job they do. They aren't just there to tell people how to eat a healthier lunch, but to ensure that all patients are given the meal plans that they require. This allows every patient to be nutritionally stable and the dietitian's work goes a long way in aiding a faster recovery and (very importantly) preventing pressure sores.

» **Physiotherapists** - once again, not every department will work alongside physiotherapists, but there are many departments that do, whether this be for chest or mobility. Physiotherapists are vital in ensuring that a patient's discharge happens promptly and smoothly, and they are masters at their work. I've witnessed chest physiotherapy send a patient's oxygen saturations from 91% to 98%, simply with some swift percussion - it's like magic!

>> **Porters** – these are the glue holding the hospital together; they do all of the day-to-day collecting and transferring of patients, they take away broken equipment and return it when it is fixed and they are always on hand to bring us anything we need (within reason – unfortunately they can't bring food). Porters are extremely important in ensuring that everything within the hospital runs smoothly, and they must build up a very impressive step count!

>> **Domestic workers** – domestic workers are another integral part of the hospital service. They ensure that the whole building is clean and infection-free, and that the ward areas are safe for everyone. They are always on hand if there is any kind of spillage and are willing to help wherever possible with a smile on their face.

>> **Play specialists** – these are generally only seen on Children's wards, where they are the eyes and ears, but that doesn't mean that they can't be called upon by anyone within the hospital. Play specialists play a vital part in ensuring the patients have the most positive experience they can have, and are always on hand to assist with distraction for difficult tasks such as taking blood or giving an injection. Although they are based on children's wards, most are more than happy to lend a hand anywhere that they are needed, such as outpatients, A&E or even on adult wards – I've known our play specialist to go to a surgical ward to help an extremely needle-phobic elderly person, so if you're ever in need of one, try phoning them. They are more than willing to help anyone who needs them and are amazing at ensuring patients have a positive experience.

Regardless of your job role, it is important to understand that everyone's contribution is vital and we can't do a good job without the help and support of the teams mentioned above. If you can respect all of your colleagues regardless of their grade or speciality, then you will maintain a positive relationship and work together effectively.

Working alongside other departments

As highlighted above, nurses are often working alongside other departments or teams.

Different departments have different pressures and priorities, so this doesn't always run as smoothly as we would like, but having a positive relationship with our colleagues in other units is a good place to start.

Working closely alongside other departments can be difficult if you don't understand the different pressures, so team building between units can be just as important as within your own team. If you are new it is a good idea to take time to explore each different department and learn how they run. This will give you an insight into the reasons they work in that way and an understanding of what they might need from you, as well as helping you to see things a little differently. This will improve your relationship greatly.

> ❝ I admire anyone who works in A&E - it is a highly pressurised environment and I know I couldn't do it. Working in paediatrics the turnover of patients is high, so we work closely alongside A&E, having frequent admissions. Communication with A&E staff is generally very good and we have a positive relationship with the nurses there. They have a great deal of pressure in their department, which can be hard to understand with little experience in this. As time has progressed, I've learned more about why they work the way they do and can understand the reasons for the decisions they have to make. One of my closest friends works in the A&E department of our hospital, so she has helped me to understand more about the way they work and I feel that I have a better relationship with the nurses there because of this. ❞

Although there can be times when two departments don't see eye to eye, it is important to remember that the priority for both will always be the patient; as long as they are getting the treatment they need, nothing else should matter. It is for this reason that it is so important to build a good relationship with the people from other departments, and you will find that it is a lot easier to work alongside people who you get on well with. Here are four things you can do to maintain a good relationship with your colleagues in other departments:

» Always be friendly - this one goes without saying, but if you are friendly and approachable towards your colleagues they are instantly more inclined to be friendly back.

» If you don't understand something, ask - if something has been done and you are not sure why, ask the nurses to explain the reason to you. As long as you are not rude about this, you won't offend them. They will be happy to explain things to you and in turn, you'll learn something new.

» Offer to help – if you know their department is extremely busy and yours isn't, check if there is anything you can do to help them with something. They will be extremely grateful for this and your relationship will improve greatly.

» Be understanding – your colleagues will never do something without good reason, so whether you can understand it or not, let it happen. As long as it doesn't jeopardise patient safety, there should be no reason to argue.

Communication

An integral part of working within a team is communication. Good communication leads to good relationships and can enable the team to remain organised and allow the working environment to run as smoothly as possible. Communication is something that we all do every day, and it's only when you stop and think about this that you realise just how important it is.

As nurses our priority is always our patient, and communication is one of the best ways to ensure that they receive the best care possible:

Communication with...	How does it help our patient?
Doctors and nurses	It allows us to keep up to date with the plan of care for our patients and ensure this is provided effectively and in a timely manner.
Members of the MDT	By communicating with other members of the MDT we can ensure that every health professional who is involved in our patient's care knows the plan and can contribute when appropriate. This in turn will help avoid delays in patient care and ensure they are discharged as soon as is possible.
Our patient and their family	Good communication with our patients has so many benefits, the most important being that: • they are aware of their plan of care, thus reducing their anxiety and ensuring that they are never left 'in the dark' • they can be given complete autonomy in the decisions regarding their care, making informed decisions wherever possible.

Nurses are constantly communicating with one another and with our patients, but we also have to communicate a great deal with other members of the multidisciplinary team. Communication between nurses is generally very good because we hand over at the start of every shift, so things are rarely missed. Communication with other teams can be more difficult, however, because we don't routinely have allotted time for this transfer of information.

If there is ever difficulty in communication (and thankfully it doesn't happen too often), it is usually between doctors and nurses; doctors are busy going from one task to another, and for most doctors if they cannot find a nurse to hand over the plan, they will document in the notes and then quickly move on to their next job. I try to make a habit of checking my patients' notes every now and then to ensure I haven't missed any changes the doctors have made. This is generally very effective, as long as their handwriting is readable!

Team building

As previously highlighted, a strong bond between team members ensures that the department runs as smoothly as possible. A great way of encouraging this bond comes through team building. This can present itself in many ways, such as working together to provide patient care at work, study days set aside specifically for team building or even meeting each other outside of work for coffee. Whichever way you develop friendships, you will become stronger as a team which in turn will ensure your patients receive the optimum care.

Functions outside of work have a great impact on the way you work as a team. When you know someone as a friend rather than a colleague, generally your relationship with that person will improve, which can help improve your ability to work well together. Whether there are two of you or twenty of you, this type of team building is crucial in enabling you and your colleagues to get to know each other better. When your colleagues are also your friends, supporting and helping one another comes naturally.

66 *When I was on my final placement I was discussing my new job with one of my mentors. The best piece of advice she gave me was to always go to social events; even if you don't know anyone, that's the way to get to know people. So that's what I*

did. On my first day I saw a poster about a birthday lunch for one of my colleagues, so I put my name down. I had never met her (and the first time I did was at the lunch) but I was assured that she wouldn't mind me going along. I'm so glad I went, because that was when I really started to get to know my colleagues. That kind of team building did wonders for me, helping my confidence improve and strengthening the bond with my work family. 🗩

To maintain a tight-knit team it is vital to create a positive working environment. Specific tasks for team building are fantastic ways to encourage a strong friendship between colleagues. These can be difficult to arrange, but can be as simple as bringing out a quick board game on a lunch break (time permitting, of course!) or arranging a nice meal (or afternoon tea, which is a favourite for myself and my colleagues). Everything you do together is team building and therefore will help to strengthen your relationships with your colleagues.

Working as a team can be difficult if morale is low. Things can happen within the team that might cause people's spirits to fall, and this can be hard to deal with. It is so much easier to work as a team when everyone is feeling positive about work, but unfortunately this is sometimes not the case. Nursing is a very difficult vocation, so it is completely understandable that people are unhappy. Below are some things you can do in your workplace to try and improve the morale for your colleagues:

» Positivity – if you can smile and stay positive, it will help your colleagues to do the same. This will boost the morale and will help to keep the friendships strong.

» Leave messages – in our staff room we have a whiteboard used for communications between the team; our manager uses it to let us know of any updates to policies, but it is also used between ourselves to communicate exciting information such as when someone has had their baby. Using this to leave messages of support is a great way to improve the morale within the team.

» Arrange social events – as previously mentioned, meeting your colleagues outside of work is a fantastic way to get to know one another. This will help to strengthen your bond as a team and will boost the team's morale greatly.

» Laugh – one of the best ways to bond as a group of friends is through laughter. When you form a friendship with your colleagues you will find it much easier to go to work and do a great job. This in turn will lead you to work extremely well together as a team, to support each other and it will greatly improve your mental wellbeing.

> 66 *Positivity is extremely important not just in work, but in day-to-day life and it's hard to stay positive when everyone else isn't feeling it. There have been times when the morale amongst my colleagues has been low, but there are amazing friendships within our team, and it's these that get us through the most difficult days. I love my team so much and I am so proud of us; we will always pull together and give our patients the best care we possibly can; and most days we can have a good laugh.* 99

Teamwork in an emergency

During an emergency situation, teamwork is particularly important. If your team is organised and you work together you can alleviate almost all of the stress from an emergency situation, thinking and acting in a logical and strategic manner that is best for both your patient and your team. Of course, it is all very well and good for me to tell you this, but when you're caught up in the moment, emergencies can be scary and frantic – especially if they are unexpected. Becoming calm and thinking logically during these situations will come with time and confidence, but working as part of an effective team can go a long way towards making these situations become far less intimidating.

Particularly when you're newly qualified, emergency situations will scare the pants off you – especially if they aren't something you see often. I'm still terrified of being in these situations; it's something that I've only been involved in once or twice and it hasn't become any less daunting. Being taught what to do is one thing, but being in that situation is another, and in that moment you will act one of two ways:

❶ You will snap into gear and know exactly what to do

OR

❷ You will freeze and wait to be given directions

Whichever of these you do will be fine – if you can stay calm and take control then that's amazing – it's something I don't think I can do (you'll have to teach me how!) but if you find yourself frozen and awaiting command, that's fine too – as long as you don't put your patient at risk. In order to ensure an emergency situation runs as smoothly as possible and to provide the best possible outcome for your patient, working within a team of people is of utmost importance. You'll have had training on emergencies as a student, and you'll definitely have more training when you start working, so I'm not going to go through the dos and don'ts – I just want to reiterate the importance of working as a team in a situation such as this.

> 66 We quite often see and treat very unwell patients who require specialist treatment that they can't always get in our district general hospital; therefore they require transfer. I'm getting used to managing and stabilising these patients with help from my colleagues, but just after my revalidation I worked a shift where there was an emergency situation that was very different to any I've been involved in before. I've had many study days in dealing with such events but when faced with a real patient, I was surprised at how unprepared I felt. I had a brief moment of thinking 'I don't know what to do!', before my instincts kicked in and I was able to assist my colleagues. Working as part of the nursing team and alongside the doctors who were also present really highlighted to me the importance of teamwork in times such as these, and the nurse in charge who was leading the situation remained extremely calm, enabling us all to do the same. The patient was very quickly stabilised and made a full recovery almost within hours, and as a team we were able to take time to discuss what happened and reflect on how well we worked together. My colleagues are an amazing group of nurses and this situation made me feel more proud of us than ever before. It is at times like these that we realise how strong our team is, and the importance of working together and supporting each other. 99

Having a supportive team is of particular importance in the aftermath of an emergency situation. Depending on the type of emergency and its outcome you might find that when you begin to reflect on the events you will need your team more than ever. Events such as these will pull you closer together and enable you to support each other through the rollercoaster of emotions you might be feeling. Having a debrief and talking things through with your colleagues is extremely important, especially with those who were also present at the time; between the team you can help establish what happened, why it happened and how you each feel about it. Don't ever shy away from these discussions, as they will help you cope with the emotions of the situation, as well as helping you to learn from the situation and gain confidence if it were to happen again.

TOP TIPS

★ Overall, working within a team is a truly wonderful experience; you will form friendships, you will help and support each other and you will ensure that your patients receive the best care possible.

★ All members of the multidisciplinary team are integral in ensuring that your patient receives holistic care that is specific to their needs. Although this might not always be plain sailing, if you can remain helpful and respectful you will be able to build a relationship of trust with everyone you work alongside.

★ Social events are great ways for you and your colleagues to get to know each other and will, in turn, help to strengthen your bond as a team. Particularly when you're new to a team, these opportunities for team building are extremely beneficial in helping you to settle in with your new work family.

★ Communication is an extremely important aspect of teamwork; good communication will ensure that your patients receive the highest quality of care possible, it will make for a smoother shift and it will greatly improve the relationships between all members of the team. When communication is poor it can cause you to spend unnecessary time chasing other teams to find out the plan of care; time which could be much better spent with your patient, building a relationship and providing this care.

★ When in an emergency situation, you will witness your team truly pulling together to work effectively for the patient in need. Although at the time this can be very scary, as long as you stay focused and think logically, you will be able to help your patient in the best way that you can. A productive debrief at the end of an emergency will also allow the team to pull together and as a group you can reflect on the events. This will both help improve the way you work together in the future, and help you on a personal level to reflect and to understand the events that have happened.

PATIENT RELATIONSHIPS

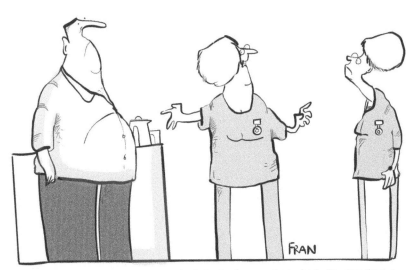

It's important to treat ALL patients as individuals. This for example is individual No. 234/98cb-k

Caring for our patients is the single most important thing that we do at work, and it is extremely important that we can begin and maintain a relationship of trust with our patients and their families. This chapter will highlight the importance of the therapeutic relationship that we build – it will explore the ways in which we can build these relationships and the positive effect they have on both our patients and ourselves. I will offer advice for those times when we struggle to build this relationship for whatever reason, and discuss the importance of setting a professional boundary both during work and outside of work, particularly regarding the use of social media.

Patient care can be a difficult subject to discuss, so before I start this chapter I will apologise if anything I'm telling you sounds bossy – I will try not to get on my high horse too much, and of course every patient is different so not everything I say here will apply to absolutely every situation. Conversely, when I find myself being too overbearing I tend to try to lighten the mood with humour, so if you find I'm trying to make light of any situation, it's only so I don't sound too overbearing, not because I don't take this topic seriously – patient care is the single most important part of nursing.

Therapeutic relationship

The term 'therapeutic relationship' is commonly used when discussing the relationship between a patient and a healthcare professional. This relationship is one of mutual trust, respect and understanding and is extremely beneficial for both parties. In children's nursing a commonly used term is 'family-centred care'; the principle here is the same as a 'therapeutic relationship', but applied to the family unit as a whole, rather than just the patient.

An essential part of this relationship must be the understanding that your patient is a person. They have lives, hobbies, families; they have life experience behind them and the person that you see in the hospital bed is only a fraction of the person that they are. It is vital to bear this in mind when forming a relationship with your patient and you must remember to treat them as a whole person, not just a condition or illness. This is easy to forget sometimes (especially if you work in a very matter-of-fact manner) and it's something that I'm making a very conscious effort to do. When discussing a patient, even if you're not near them, always make an effort to refer to them by name, not bed number or condition. For example, instead of saying "the chest infection in bed 4" say "Steve in bed 4, with a chest infection".

Saying that, in this chapter I will always refer to patients as 'patients', despite highlighting that they are people. This is essentially because saying 'people' too much can get very confusing.

I'll stop the lecture here, and on we get with *Chapter Three*.

Building relationships

If you are a clinical nurse, working with patients is something you will be doing day in and day out; it's what you go to work for. If your work setting doesn't have a high turnover of patients (or even if it does), you will get to know every one of the patients you care for and you will begin a therapeutic relationship with all of them. You might become closer to some than others; this is human nature, but everyone you care for will leave something with you – I can still remember the first patient I met on my first day as a student nurse.

As nurses, we have the unique and wonderful opportunity to build relationships with our patients; we can get to know them and their families, build relationships with them and know that we have made a positive impact on their lives. This is the most rewarding aspect of nursing and it is the reason that we chose this vocation. Forming relationships with our patients is a wonderful thing to do; it provides them with someone to talk to when there might be no one else, it allows us to learn about their lives and can even change our perspective about the world. As a nurse, it is the greatest feeling to know that we have made a positive impact on the lives of our patients and their families.

Different nurses will have conflicting opinions about how much it is appropriate to bond with our patients; some might prefer to remain strictly professional while others like to have a chat and get to know the people we are caring for. No matter which of these stances you adopt, it is important to ensure that your patient is happy with the relationship you have formed and is comfortable - don't try to be overly chatty with a patient who doesn't want this, but equally, if your patient is worried or scared, being open and forming a relationship will greatly help ease their worries.

There are many reasons that we might form a bond with our patients, for example:

» We might share something in common with them.

» They might have a particularly sad background.

» They might be with us for a long time and we get to know them well.

» They might remind us of someone.

» It simply happens for an unknown reason.

Whatever the reason we form a connection with these patients, it is important to remember that there are boundaries and that we must not treat any patient differently - I will explore this more as the chapter progresses.

Having something in common with a patient instantly provides us with a great starting point in striking a positive relationship. It gives you a topic for discussion and immediately puts both you and your patient at ease. This could be anything from supporting the same sports team, enjoying the same music or even watching the same TV programmes - anything that will provide you with a talking point. When you build this positive rapport with a patient your relationship with them will thrive, and you'll create an extremely positive experience for both them and their family.

When you have this talking point, your patient might find it easier to open up to you, they will be more willing to take on your advice where needed and, most importantly, it will give them company in an otherwise very lonely environment. This is hugely beneficial to them (and you) for many reasons which will be explored later in this chapter.

Sometimes, we bond with patients because they have a particularly sad background. They might have a terminal or life-limiting illness, they might have no family to visit them or the circumstances of their admission might be upsetting. For example, in paediatrics, we sometimes have children admitted to the ward as a place of safety if there are safeguarding concerns. Patients such as these have a tendency to pull on our heartstrings and allow us the ability to form bonds unlike those with some other patients. You will very often witness a change in their character and personality as they grow more confident around the hospital team and in turn you might grow closer to them. It is sometimes these patients who are the hardest to care for, particularly if they affect you in this way. When they are then discharged it can evoke a strange feeling of sadness, or even guilt, and it is more important than ever to remember the boundaries that must be set within a therapeutic patient relationship.

> 66 *I sometimes find it hard not to become emotionally invested with a patient or family, and in cases such as child protection concerns it becomes even more of a challenge. One patient who stands out in my mind was admitted under these circumstances and on the ward for around a week. During this time we built a relationship with the child, getting to know them and helping them trust our team, but after an extensive investigation by social services they were then discharged home - back into the environment that they had come from. At first I found it very difficult to feel anything but guilt because I had seen how much the patient had flourished in the short time they were with us. However, after talking things through with the safeguarding team I learned that it is important to trust the decisions made by these professionals, even if you don't feel they're right at the time. The patient has thrived since their discharge home and there have been no other concerns.* 99

On every ward there will be patients who have either been with you for an extended period of time, or who are 'frequent flyers' (patients who have had numerous previous admissions) so it is very likely that you will take care of them often and be given the opportunity to get to know them and their families well. As you spend time with them you will learn about their lives and this is a wonderful way of building a positive relationship with them. It will help them to trust you and with time your relationship will become stronger and more positive. These patients almost become 'part of the furniture' of the ward, and it can feel strange when they are then discharged.

Possibly the most emotionally provoking reason that we become close to a patient is that they remind us of someone. Whether this is a loved one, a friend or even someone from the television, these patients will already have made an impact on us from the very start and can give us mixed emotions depending on who it is that they remind us of. We can either form a close bond with them or we can find it difficult to keep a professional distance, purely because they evoke our emotions. Maintaining this professional boundary can be one of the hardest aspects of the job.

> 66 As a student nurse my first placement was on an adult ward. I loved that placement and very nearly changed my speciality to adult nursing; however, there is one very important reason that I didn't, and that was because I found it too sad. I felt that almost every elderly patient I cared for reminded me of one of my grandparents, and I couldn't have coped with that day in and day out. One patient I still think about to this day is a lovely gentleman who reminded me so much of my Grandpa in his mannerisms. I was able to spend time with him and developed a very positive relationship with him, and he was the first person I gave an injection to (he told me I was very gentle). He was discharged early into my placement and seeing him go home was very bittersweet for me – I then realised that I couldn't work on an adult ward. Some of my friends who are adult nurses tell me that they don't know how I work on a children's ward as they'd find it 'too sad', but I feel exactly the same about adult nursing; I just couldn't do it. Hats off to all you wonderful adult nurses out there! 99

Sometimes, we don't know the reason that we form a bond with a particular patient; it just happens. You might find that it takes something in particular such as a procedure that you're helping with, and sometimes you might instantly 'click' and form an immediate rapport. It is patients such as these who are my favourite to care for, as the therapeutic relationship of trust is created almost instantly and you immediately know that you're making a difference in the lives of these families.

> 66 Not long after I'd qualified I nursed a girl who had broken her arm and needed surgery for this, so was admitted during the night shift. I was on the following day and when I introduced myself I knew that I would form a positive relationship with this family. The girl was with her mum, dad and older brother and the family dynamic was like nothing I'd seen before – you could tell that everyone adored each other and had exactly the same sense of humour; it was amazing to watch. Throughout the course of the day I got to know this family extremely well, and I actually felt sad when my shift ended and I had to say goodbye to them. I don't know what it was that made me click so well with this family but I'm so glad that I did, and I still think of them to this day. 99

Every patient that you care for will have an impact on you in some way, and no matter what the circumstances of their admission or the reason that your relationship is built, you will enjoy getting to know the family and making a positive impact on their lives.

Boundaries

Forming a relationship of trust with your patient and their family is hugely beneficial for many reasons; however, it is extremely important to maintain boundaries in these situations. There is a fine line between being friendly and being friends, and sometimes it can be hard to distinguish this. It's great to have a good relationship with your patient and their family, but as a nurse you must always remain professional. Knowing when you're close to the 'line' can sometimes be difficult; what might be a normal conversation for one family might become too much information to another, so you will have to use your own judgement of each family to decide upon your own boundaries with them.

In order to ensure your safety as well as your patient's, the boundary must always be set by yourself as the nurse, never by your patient or their family. Ensuring that you don't 'cross a line' with a patient can become difficult when they want to become more friendly than you are comfortable with. An example of this might be a discussion with a patient where they ask you for information about yourself that you deem to be too intimate or personal. If this does happen to you, give them very vague information, or tell them politely that you aren't comfortable with the conversation and try to change the subject. If they are persistent you should speak to the nurse in charge or your line manager regarding their conduct and they can advise you as to what you can do in the situation. It might be an idea for the nurse in charge to re-allocate the patient to another nurse so that they cannot continue to push boundaries with you.

In the same way, be aware of your colleagues and whether their patients are attempting to get too personal with them. As highlighted in the previous chapter, teamwork is essential within nursing and your colleagues rely on you as much as you rely on them. If you do notice that a patient is becoming too friendly with a colleague, or vice versa, you should highlight this to both your colleague and the nurse in charge, for the same reasons as above. Your colleague's safety is as important as your own, and, of course, your patient's.

If you find it difficult to know where you should set the boundaries in your relationship with your patient, this list of important factors will help. However, every patient is different so your relationship with them will also be different. Your own judgement will be your best indicator of where this line must be set, but these top tips are important to remember.

» This goes without saying, but it is a very important one – you must absolutely never enter a romantic or sexual relationship with a patient or their relative.

» Second to that, forming a friendship with a client can also become tricky business and should never be done, particularly if they have been a 'long-termer' or 'frequent flyer'. Socialising outside of work with a patient can open a can of worms and can cause you a conflict of interest; it can become difficult to maintain a nurse/patient relationship if you strike a true friendship with a patient. We are all human so it is possible that you might feel yourself getting too friendly with a patient or their family, but in every circumstance it is up to you to put your professional conduct first.

» Another one that should go without saying, but is becoming an increasing problem within nursing (so much so that there's a section

45

on it later in this chapter) is the use of social media. To put it briefly – don't accept a patient's friend request, ensure your privacy is turned up and don't put anything on there about a patient or your work.

» When chatting to a patient, it's fine to tell them a little about yourself in order to establish your professional relationship, but once this rapport is formed, there is no need to go any further. For example it's nice to chat about your children, but they don't need to know your son's pet rat's birthday (I know this sounds a little over the top, and of course it's all in jest, but you'd be surprised).

» The subject of accepting gifts from patients can become difficult, largely because there are multiple schools of thought and it relies on perspective. The NMC Code of Conduct states that nurses should accept only trivial gifts, in order to avoid the perception that a nurse is being 'bribed' to provide better care to some patients than others. I know that I wouldn't change my care based on something such as this, and I like to think no other nurses would, but of course we have to be careful. For this one you can almost certainly use your common sense; in short, accepting a box of chocolates is fine, but if the patient tries to give you the keys to their Ferrari, you're better off politely declining their generous offer.

» Conversely, you shouldn't buy gifts for your patient either. There might be small exceptions here, for example if we have children with birthdays on our ward we will give them something small from the team as a whole, but buying personal gifts for patients can be seen as favouritism and should be avoided.

A positive relationship

As previously mentioned, building a positive relationship with patients is hugely beneficial to both yourself and your patients for a number of reasons:

Benefits for the patient	Benefits for the nurse
• Being a patient can be lonely, but having a good relationship with the nurses goes a long way towards helping patients to feel comfortable and cared for.	• When you're having a busy day, developing a good relationship with your patients will help you to see the good in what you're doing and really improve your outlook.

Benefits for the patient	Benefits for the nurse
• If the patient has a positive relationship with their healthcare professional they will in turn have a positive overall experience of their hospital stay. For vulnerable patients, children or 'frequent flyers' this can help alleviate fear of hospitals or the stress of a possible re-admission. • Patients who trust their nurses are more likely to open up about certain aspects of their care; for example, they might previously have been afraid to speak out against a doctor or plan of care, but will trust you enough to inform you. This means that you can then voice their concerns and ensure they receive the appropriate care. • We've all nursed patients who think that they know best, but by building a relationship of mutual trust and respect they are more likely to take on board the advice they are given and act upon it. This will in turn help their condition improve more quickly and make their stay shorter.	• As a nurse, knowing that you're providing the best care possible gives you incredible job satisfaction. • Patients who are open with you are a lot less mentally challenging than those who aren't, and when they are open and honest with you it becomes far easier to provide the best care for their needs. • Your day will run much more smoothly if you and your patient are both working together to achieve the best care. In the same way, if you don't see eye to eye with your patient it can become very difficult to move forward.

❝ I recently worked a shift that was extremely busy, with each of my patients requiring a slightly higher level of care than usual. At the end of this shift, although I was exhausted, I felt very happy and came home smiling. This can sometimes be very unusual for me (mainly because I get grumpy when I'm tired), but on this occasion every patient and parent that I was caring for was lovely, making it impossible for me to think I'd had a bad day. I built very strong relationships with the patients I was caring for, and they were open and honest with me about every aspect of their care; if they didn't think something was right, they'd tell me and we would work out a different way to do it. Although I was busy I knew that I was providing the best care I possibly could for each of my patients, and it's on days such as those that I really love being a nurse – even if it does take at least 12 hours of sleep to recover. ❞

Establishing a good relationship

As previously noted, when you've built a rapport with your patients the experience becomes so much more positive for both parties. Establishing this relationship can be difficult at times, so here are a few handy hints on how to achieve this on your initial meeting:

» Introduce yourself – this should be the first thing that you do when you meet your patient. You might have seen the #hellomynameis campaign floating around, and this is an extremely good way of reminding us of the importance of our initial meeting. For example, my usual introduction goes something like this: *big welcoming smile* "Hello, my name is Lauren, I'm one of the nurses on the ward and I'll be looking after you today. If you need anything at all just let me know, but I'll be in and out anyway." (or "You've got me again!" if I've looked after them on the previous day). This way my patient knows my name and role and can begin to trust me instantly.

» Ask them their preferred name – when nursing adults in particular, this will definitely go a long way in helping you to show your respect for your patient; for example "Hello Mrs Smith, is that what you'd like me to call you?" This will immediately help your patient feel at ease and will show that you care about them.

» If they have a parent or relative with them, ask them their names too. This is something I didn't do when I first qualified, but one day I was working with a student nurse and felt almost ashamed when she asked the patient's mum her name and shook her hand – I couldn't believe that I'd never thought to do this before! It will really go a long way in promoting the therapeutic relationship and shows that you care for the whole family unit, not just the patient.

» Ask if you can get them anything – who doesn't love a cuppa first thing in the morning? (or evening if you're on the night shift). Offer to get them some tea, or ask if they're hungry or need pain relief. This will immediately help them feel comfortable and you'll have a good relationship for the rest of the shift – especially if you bring them tea.

» Always be cheery – a big smile goes a long way!

These things may seem trivial to you, but to your patient and their relatives they will go a long way in reassuring them that they are in safe hands. Making a good first impression is extremely important, but keeping this up is equally so. It is vital that throughout your patient's time in hospital they see you as someone they can trust, and therefore you must always remain their advocate, no matter what the doctors or other care providers have decided for them.

> 66 When working alongside doctors, I am always aware that I might be the strongest advocate for my patient. Some patients or parents are almost 'scared' of doctors and don't want to speak against them or the decisions they have made, leaving it to the nursing team to discuss this. It's quite common for patients or parents to nod along with the doctor while they are being assessed, and when the doctor leaves they explode into panic because they didn't understand what was being said. When I know a doctor has spoken to my patient I will always speak to them after, ensuring that they understand exactly what they have been told, and I always ask if they have any questions. This way I know that they are happy with the plan of care and parents are usually much more comfortable discussing this with me than the doctors. 99

There is more information on establishing and maintaining a good relationship in *Chapter Four: Difficult situations* - look under the heading 'Uncooperative patients'. Although this is about a different topic, the content still stands.

What if I don't strike a relationship with a patient?

There might be times where it is difficult to build a rapport with your patient, which can happen for any number of reasons. Some patients might wish to have a strictly professional relationship with their healthcare workers, while other patients might be shy, or not used to having someone to talk to, so they might struggle when faced with this new experience. These patients might need to take a little time to open up and be able to fully trust you. There are ways that you can attempt to establish this rapport if you think your patient would benefit from it, and if they are shy you'll provide them with a talking point that might be a great way to bring them out of their shell.

» Ask them about their lives - you'll need to use your judgement as to whether your patient will be comfortable telling you about themselves, but most people are more than happy to share stories about their life or tell you all about their wonderful children/grandchildren/friends. This will show them that you are genuinely interested in them as a person, not just as a patient.

» Take an interest in what they are doing - hospitals can be boring, so often patients might be reading a book or magazine, playing a game on their phone or working through a puzzle book. Whatever they are doing, taking an interest in this will provide you with a talking point and can help to establish a great rapport.

» Ask them about something topical - is Christmas approaching? Ask if they're ready; what they've asked Santa for; what they've bought for their relative who visited this morning. Is it lunch time? Ask about their favourite foods or whether they like to cook. What's been in the news recently? Ask their opinions on the events; chat about the world. There are so many topics you can talk about, so choose one and start chatting; you can move on to another if they have nothing to say.

> 66 I really love getting to know my patients and their families when they come into the ward. I always try to stay cheerful (as long as the circumstances allow) and when I know the family will take it well, I'll say things like "holler if you need anything!" before I leave their room. When you can get to know the people individually it makes the job so much more enjoyable, and I once had a dad peer around the curtain, see me walking past and shout 'Holler' at the top of his voice. It's times like these that being a nurse is really wonderful - you get to know the people you're caring for and can really form a relationship of trust and respect with them. 99

However, human nature dictates that we won't always strike a relationship with everyone; in the same way we can 'click' with someone for an unknown reason, we can also 'clash' with others. If there is a specific patient you haven't connected with, don't try to force it; we will all form different types of relationships with different people. Of course, always give every patient the same level of care, but on a personal level, don't worry if you get along with one person better than another. If you find that you haven't 'hit it off' with a patient straight away, you can be safe in the knowledge that they will still have a positive experience from the great quality of care you've provided them.

If there is a patient or relative that you don't agree with, always remember that your opinion should absolutely not affect the care you provide; just because you disagree with someone does not mean that they are a bad person or that they deserve any less compassionate care than the patient in the next bed. If you find it incredibly difficult to care for someone in this way, speak to the nurse in charge and see if they can reallocate the patient to another nurse. This will be expanded further in the next chapter, but don't feel too guilty if this does happen, as some personalities do clash; the important thing to remember is that the patient care should never ever suffer.

Social media

Possibly one of the most prominent subjects of our day and age is related to social media – that was my first ever lecture at university, even before "welcome to uni!". Social media is a wonderful thing when used correctly; it allows us to keep in touch with old friends who we don't necessarily see very often, it allows us to share our stories and experiences with loved ones and it allows us to meet new people and learn from them.

However, it is also a topic that we need to approach very sensibly and I can't stress enough the importance of upholding a professional reputation both inside and outside of work. The amount of NMC hearings regarding social media is ever increasing, so please be extremely careful with what you post online.

There are more and more social media sites becoming available, including (but not limited to):

» Facebook

» Twitter

» Photo sites such as Instagram or Flickr

» Tumblr

» Blogging sites such as blogspot or wordpress

» LinkedIn.

It's fine to use these websites, but always be wary of what you're posting and who you're friends with on them. You could get into serious trouble if you use them incorrectly, and it's really not worth losing your job over. Below is a list of some Dos and Don'ts of social media. Once again, sorry if I come across as bossy and overbearing, but this is such an important topic.

Dos	Don'ts
• Always be aware of what you're posting, who can see it and what it says about you as a professional. Also remember, any future employers might search for you, so make sure they are not put off by what you've posted.	• Under no circumstances should you become friends with a patient or their relative. This is a big no-no – if they request to be your friend, don't accept it, no matter how well you know them, and never ever send a friend request to them.
• Turn your privacy settings way up and ensure that anyone who isn't your friend or follower can see only the bare minimum.	• Avoid posting pictures or statuses that could undermine your professional image, such as photos when drunk, or material that is derogatory or contains innuendo.
• Only post important topics that are personal to you, keep them professional and meaningful. Always think about your image and what your social media account says about you.	• Don't 'air your dirty laundry' all over the internet. Keep it between whoever is involved; the whole world doesn't want to know about your argument with your neighbour.
• It's fine to follow pages or sites that are related to your job; for example, if your hospital has a Facebook page, it's fine to follow this, but again, be aware of who can see your comments. It's up to us all to ensure nurses have a good reputation in the public eye.	• Never post confidential information regarding a patient, colleague or your work, including photos. Also, never use it to intimidate or bully your colleagues (or anyone for that matter).
• Use social media to help build your relationship with your colleagues and other nurses around the world – you can learn a lot from others, but restrict this to the specific groups only, and not publicly – I'll expand further below.	• Avoid commenting on public posts where possible, especially if your profile shows that you are a nurse. For example, if a news website posts about a topic that you comment on, ensure that your comment is respectful and professional because anyone can click on your profile and see where you work.

Dos	Don'ts
• Be sensible – I'm not telling you to come off social media completely and live like a hermit, but just use common sense about what you're posting and who can see it.	• Don't phone in sick for work and then post pictures of yourself in a bar or out with friends; that will definitely get you in trouble.

There are fantastic benefits that can arise from the use of social media. For example, the hospital I work for has its own Facebook and Twitter pages which they use to promote the amazing work being done by the different teams within the Trust. They promote specific events such as fundraising and they also highlight problems or raise awareness. On several occasions they have posted about the A&E department becoming overwhelmed with patients who do not necessarily need to attend A&E and advise alternative ways to get checked out. These are always met with a wonderful response from the public and within a few hours the department has become manageable again. In this way, social media is really amazing.

One of the reasons I love social media is that you can communicate with other nurses and professionals who work in your field. This can be done in a variety of ways; for example there are private Facebook groups, such as the Royal College of Nursing Students page which I have found extremely helpful over the years. Here, you can post privately about comments or questions regarding nursing matters and provide others with reassurance if they have worries or concerns. Another amazing group of people are those who run the Twitter page @WeNurses and their sub-groups. These pages hold regular weekly chats and allow nurses around the country to join in discussions about the various topical events and allow anyone to share their experiences (within reason). They are extremely supportive to anyone out there asking for help and the community will rally around to provide help and guidance where possible.

> 66 I always try to be sensible about what I post on Facebook and Twitter, and I'm growing more aware of what is deemed to be acceptable and what isn't. I will never post anything about work, or whether I've had a bad day; however, when I've had a great day I do sometimes mention a vague post about

how much I love my job (but never go into detail or mention specifics). As a student I think I talked about placements more than I do now, although never said anything that would get me into trouble – I paid attention in that lecture! You will always hear horror stories about nurses who have been struck off the NMC register for misuse of social media, and these stories have been enough to scare me from posting anything work-related. In this section I promise I am not trying to scare you off social media, because I also use it to speak to other nurses and join in discussions as highlighted above and find these so helpful and thought-provoking. I just really want people to be more aware of what is being posted on their accounts and who can see it. **99**

TOP TIPS

★ It is so important that we create a therapeutic relationship of trust with our patients to ensure that they receive the best care possible, and to allow them to be comfortable enough to be open and honest with us during times when decisions about their care must be made. Having this relationship is so important both for our patients and for ourselves, therefore it is vital that we establish this as early on as possible.

★ There are many reasons that this relationship is made; sometimes this is because we simply 'click', other times it will take a particular event happening. Every patient is different, so our relationship with them will be different; the most important thing to remember is that we must not treat one patient differently to any other, regardless of the relationship we have built.

★ There are times when for whatever reason we do not click with our patients, but this doesn't mean that we never will. Some people need time before they can grow to trust you, so it is important that you allow them this time. Some patients will be more open with you than others, and some might take time to get to know you before they fully trust you. As long as you remain respectful and caring, your patient will grow to trust you in time, and even if they never do, you will know that you have provided them with the best care that you possibly can.

★ Setting boundaries with your patients is an essential aspect of building this therapeutic relationship, and it is done subconsciously in almost every case. Although it doesn't happen often, there can be times when our patients might try to push these boundaries or become too over-friendly. It is important that this be highlighted as early as possible and that the patients (or nurses) know when they have pushed the boundaries, but this must be done as politely as possible – some people might not realise when they are becoming too friendly.

★ Social media is one of the most important things to be mindful of, and it is increasingly becoming more so. Nursing is a professional vocation, and this professionalism must be reflected both inside and outside of work. Always keep in mind what your social media account says about you; turn your privacy settings all the way up, and under no circumstances should you ever post anything about work or a patient – you never know who will be able see it.

DIFFICULT SITUATIONS

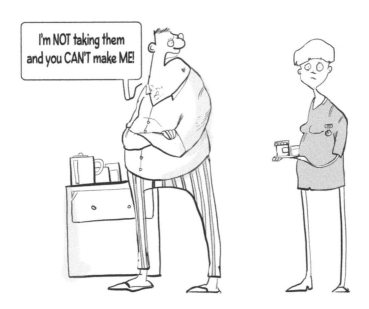

Nursing isn't always easy and for many different reasons we can find ourselves faced with difficult situations. I am determined that this chapter will not be downbeat, but my aim here is to be honest about some events that might happen to you at some point along the way. This chapter will discuss the ways in which our patients can have an emotional effect on us in many different ways, such as if they are in pain, if we have to break bad news or when our patient has died. I will explore the best ways to cope with patients who are aggressive or uncooperative and will explore basic principles of conflict resolution. I will briefly look into other ways that nursing can be difficult, such as through 'work politics' or through having disagreements with colleagues, and will discuss what happens if you or your colleague makes a mistake at work.

It is important to point out here that this chapter contains a lot of patient stories, so to protect patient confidentiality some details such as age, gender or illness have been changed.

Emotional difficulties

Patients can be a source of difficulty to us for a number of reasons, and possibly the hardest thing can be seeing a patient suffering or in pain. This isn't something that you will necessarily get used to, even as the years go on. Not all patients will affect us in the same way (see *Chapter Three*), but there are some who do affect us, and this can make our job particularly difficult. To be a nurse you need to have a unique balance of both compassion and hardiness; we can't be upset all the time about our patients, but we can't be robots either. It's a fine line and there will be instances when our patients will pull on our heartstrings.

It's not nice to see anyone suffering (that's the reason I don't often watch the news!) and when your patient is suffering in front of you it becomes one of the hardest aspects of nursing. I am getting better at this than when I first began my training, but I'd never say it doesn't bother me. Whatever your speciality, there will be something that you're better at coping with, for example nursing children doesn't often upset me whereas the thought of nursing elderly people does. Others might really enjoy nursing older people, but find the thought of nursing children upsetting.

> 66 *I don't often get upset when looking after children because there is always a light at the end of the tunnel; I know they'll be back to their normal cheeky selves soon, but there will always be times when something pulls on my heartstrings. There is one particular little person who does this every time: a gorgeous little boy with a degenerative illness. From the time of his diagnosis to the time I am writing this he has gone downhill quickly - the first time I met him he was active and chatty, now he is confined to a wheelchair and unable to communicate. His family are truly amazing and their relationship with our nursing team is wonderful. The hardest time for me when caring for him was shortly after he lost the ability to talk. He was getting ready to go home (which was brilliant, of course) so I removed his cannula, but as I looked up at him I saw one solitary tear roll down his face. This absolutely broke my heart because I knew he couldn't communicate to me that it was hurting him. He is a little fighter though and is doing extremely well!* 99

It is common that we will encounter these emotional difficulties during our work - after all, we are all human - so there is nothing wrong with letting it affect us. Everyone copes with this differently; some people switch off emotionally, others have a good cry and let it all out. You will find your own way to deal with these feelings, but if you're struggling you'll find some tips that can help at the end of the chapter.

Uncooperative patients

As nurses we can sometimes find ourselves trying to provide treatment or care to patients who are unwilling to cooperate. Depending on the setting you work in, you might experience this more than others, for example patients with mental health problems might be typically more uncooperative than those without. As a children's nurse (and I'm sure any parents out there can back me up on this), there are many times where I have found myself trying to bargain with a tiny person in order for them to take their medicine; sometimes you win and sometimes you lose. I'd be lying if I said this was my favourite aspect of my job, but it is sometimes nice to see their true personalities come out.

This can, however, become very difficult for several reasons; for example, your patient might be refusing treatment that you know will benefit them, which can become both frustrating and upsetting. The two eventualities of this occurrence are:

you have to allow them to go without the medication

OR

you have you give it without their consent (however there are only certain occasions when this can be done)

Your patient's mental capacity and ability to give consent will determine which of these you can do:

>> If they have full capacity and are able to make an informed decision, you simply have to respect this.

>> If they have been sectioned under the Mental Health Act 1983 then they are deemed to be unable to consent for themselves and therefore you are able to give them the treatment they require, even if they refuse. However, this is only providing it is in the patient's best interest.

>> If your patient needs emergency treatment but is unable to give consent, for example they are rushed into A&E unconscious or are under general anaesthetic in theatre, you are required to give this treatment without consent, but this must be explained to the patient when possible.

» If you work with children, the general rule is that if the child is deemed Gillick competent (able to make an informed decision for themselves), they must be allowed to do so. If they are too young then the responsibility falls to their legal guardian and you're able to give medication, even if the child refuses.

The subject of consent does go a little deeper than this, but I won't cover it any further. For more information there are plenty of sources you can look at; I used the NHS Choices website (www.nhs.uk).

66 I've come across many instances where a child (usually aged 2-7) has refused to take their medication, and there is no choice other than to bargain with them, and if that doesn't work, with their parent's permission we simply force the syringe in (I promise it isn't as brutal as it sounds). This is never a nice thing to do, but I've got used to it now and we have learned the best ways to get this done as quickly as possible. It is very rare that doing this ever becomes upsetting because it is a day-to-day occurrence, but I remember one patient with a kidney condition who was refusing to take her medications. Together with the patient's family I tried to convince her to take these medicines and her mum had even attempted to hide them in her drink, but she was too clever for us and refused point blank to drink it. I'd been trying since 08.00 to convince her that she needed it and by 14.00 it was clear that it wouldn't be voluntary. We had no choice but to hold her down and give her the medication. She screamed, cried and spat, and no matter how hard we tried we could not get this into her. We eventually had to pass an NG tube and give the medication that way; I felt awful. Normally I'm not affected by this because I know it is in the child's best interest, but on this occasion I was so upset – partly because I felt like a horrible person, but also because I felt frustrated and defeated. 99

If you're nursing an adult with full capacity who is refusing treatment, I imagine this to be very difficult; particularly if you know that without it they will become very unwell. You know there is nothing you can do and that this decision must be theirs, but that doesn't stop you feeling like a bad nurse (which you're not, I promise). I sometimes don't know which would make me feel worse; pinning them down and making them take medication or having no option but to let them go without it; both eventualities place you in a very difficult situation.

If your patient is refusing a drug, don't write them off instantly as being 'awkward'; take some time to talk to them and try to find out why they don't want it. They might be worried about a side-effect, there might be a misconception surrounding the drug that they have concerns about, or if it's an injection they might simply be scared of needles. Talking to them about their concerns might make them feel a lot better or make them change their mind, but even if it doesn't you will know that you've done all you can.

Dealing with challenging people

As nurses we deal with members of the public on a day-to-day basis, and it is inevitable that we will encounter some who are more understanding than others. It is becoming increasingly common to experience some sort of hostility, violence or intimidation from patients or their relatives, and therefore it is important that as nurses we know how to keep ourselves, our colleagues and our patients safe.

There are many reasons why people become hostile towards medical professionals, and although I am by no means condoning this behaviour, it can help you to defuse the situation if you understand your patient's frustrations. The section below (mainly the right-hand column) also applies to *Chapter Three* - see the section on 'Establishing a good relationship'.

Why are they hostile?	What you can do to prevent/ relieve this
Being a patient or visitor can be very stressful; tensions run high and people tend to have a lower tolerance than they normally would. This is also the case when patients are in pain or seeing their family members in pain.	Understand that this is a stressful time for people and ensure that you are always approachable. Always be open and honest with them and try to alleviate this stress where possible. In my experience, a cup of tea works very well in certain situations, so if you judge that it will be well received, it can be a good starting point.

Why are they hostile?	What you can do to prevent/ relieve this
Waiting for answers can take time, which adds to the patient's anxiety, particularly if the possible diagnosis is a bad one.	Try to provide your patients with answers as soon as possible, even if that means telling them honestly when the results aren't back or that there has been a delay for whatever reason. Honesty really is the best policy, and your patient would rather be in the loop.
Some people might have a lack of understanding, either of the medical terminology or of the situation as a whole. This can cause extra worry or frustration, especially if their perception of the situation is that it is more serious than it is (and sometimes we nurses can be very blasé about things because we see them so often - it's easy to forget that routine things for us are terrifying to our patients).	Explain everything as simply and basically as you can; medical jargon will just confuse people and cause them to feel overwhelmed. Fact sheets are a great way to do this by allowing them to read about their condition in their own time. Offer them paper and a pen in order to jot down any questions they think of while you're not there, and where applicable, only give them the information they need to know at that time.
Patients who have had multiple admissions with few or no answers are likely to be at the end of their tether and are less likely to trust what the healthcare professionals are telling them, even if there is no cause for concern.	Trust them, even if this means you end up back where you started. Most people don't generally worry for no reason, and if they tell you something is wrong, it probably is - you don't want to take that chance. A golden rule in children's nursing is 'trust mum' - parents know their child best so if they are telling you something isn't right, nine times out of ten this is true. The same applies with adults; never make them feel that they are worrying for nothing.
Some patients might have a mental health problem which can cause them to become violent or angry.	Knowing about your patient's mental health condition and how to respond to this appropriately is important here. People with mental health problems can be unpredictable, so having good conflict resolution skills is also vital (see later in this chapter for more in-depth information regarding this).

Why are they hostile?	What you can do to prevent/ relieve this
Sometimes, you might simply find a patient who takes a dislike to you.	Sadly, if this is the case there isn't much you can do. Being extremely nice to them is usually my default setting here, mostly because I hate confrontation, but this will generally go one of two ways: 1) they'll be fine with me or 2) they won't. Try and judge how you think they'll respond and act accordingly. My advice here would be: don't let them get to you, don't rise to them, and most importantly, and I can't stress this enough, **don't treat them any differently than you would any other patient**.

66 *Thankfully, *touch wood* I've never been involved in a situation where a parent or patient has become physically violent, although I have known it to happen. I have, however, been in many situations where a parent has become very verbally aggressive towards me or my colleagues, and this can be very difficult to deal with. It used to really upset me and I'd take it to heart, but I'm now beginning to harden to it and understand the reasons why people get so frustrated. I would never let it change my practice though, and I still treat those patients the same way I would anyone else (although I am happier to see them leave than some others). Unfortunately, it's becoming more part of the job and we just have to learn to deal with it and leave it behind us - that's the hard bit.* 99

Conflict resolution is a mandatory skill that is taught in most (if not all) Trusts, so you'll definitely be trained in this within your first few weeks. It was taught to us in university and was part of the induction process when I started my job, so it is something that I will always remember as being very important. I won't delve too deeply into it, but the main aim of conflict resolution is preventing a situation from escalating. This is done by becoming more aware of our body language and tone of voice.

Here are five key points to remember:

>> Remain calm and adopt an 'open' stance

>> Never rise to someone or argue back – this will cause the situation to escalate quickly

>> You are permitted to use minimal force, but only if this is reasonable and required – don't hit out if there is another way around it

>> Always remain near the door and never let yourself be backed into a corner

>> Get out and get help if you're worried a situation is escalating – there is safety in numbers so if possible, try and find backup.

By following these tips you can help ensure your safety and that of your patients. If you are in this situation you must escalate it as per your Trust guidelines; for example, call security to remove the person (if appropriate) and report it using your incident reporting system.

Politics

No matter where you go or what you do there will always be politics – it's inevitable, and nursing is no different. Wherever you work there will always be an element of political unrest, which can be caused by the UK government, the senior Trust management, your immediate manager or your colleagues on the 'shop floor'. Unfortunately, that is the way nursing is, and there isn't a great deal that you can do about it. Don't worry, this section isn't my way of throwing my political preferences at you and I will try to withhold my opinion here as much as possible. The purpose of this section is simply to tell you of my experiences and maybe offer a little help if you can relate to any of them.

In my experience, the main causes of political unease within nursing are because of the following issues:

>> Pay – this issue is something that has been going on for years, and is still at the forefront of the nursing agenda. This one shouldn't cause too much disruption when you're on the shop floor, but it is causing a lot of nurses to struggle. Working harder for less pay is something that will get you down over time but try not to let it affect the way you work, and remember: you're in this job because you care, not for the money.

>> Paperwork – the amount of paperwork that we have to do is ever-increasing, and sometimes it really does feel like we do more paperwork than patient care. The NMC Code offers advice regarding record keeping so I won't go into that here.

I definitely understand the reasons that paperwork is important; we always strive to do the best thing for our patients. Good documentation allows for better communication between the MDT and promotes patient safety and continuity of care. It is also important for us as nurses – today's culture means that we might need to cover our backs in the event of a complaint or error; **if it isn't documented, it didn't happen**. However, there are times when I can't help but feel that I spend more time filling in documentation than with my patients, which can be difficult. If there is an emergency situation, however, I make notes as I go and then document in retrospect. Documentation will always come second to patient care in instances such as these, and to be fair, I don't know anyone who wouldn't do this: patient care is ALWAYS our priority.

> 66 *Some of my colleagues have been working for a long time, and I love hearing about how different nursing was when they first started. I am amazed by the amount that they were able to do in terms of workload and patient care – I can't imagine being able to fit it all in, particularly back in the days when parents were only allowed to visit at specific times. But there is one main difference between then and now, and that is the paperwork. They all agree that there was far less 'back then', and I don't know if there were ever any repercussions from this. One thing they all agree on is that nursing is changing, and you have to move with it otherwise you will become extremely unhappy.* 99

>> Staffing and Workload – these are possibly the most encountered problems in the nursing climate and ones that can be very difficult to deal with, especially when you're newly qualified or lack confidence. When your colleagues are also extremely busy it leaves little time for you to support each other. Having a heavy workload is still something that I struggle with a great deal, especially when we are short-staffed. In nursing, it is definitely a fact that no two days are the same and there are many affecting factors; you can have one day where you are fully staffed and have a steady patient

workload, followed by a day with a colleague off sick and a higher acuity of patients. This can be very difficult to cope with, and I will expand on this in *Chapter Five*. If you're struggling with a particularly heavy workload my main piece of advice to you is to just do what you can. You're (probably) not a superhero; you can't do absolutely everything so just do the utmost that you can and you'll have done enough. Don't let it get you down - you're brilliant!

In *Chapter Two* I mentioned how difficult it can be to work as part of a team when the morale is low, and these 'political' problems can be a cause of this. You're never going to be working with a group of people who are entirely happy all the time, but you won't get anywhere if you let it get you down. The main thing to remember is that it absolutely mustn't affect the way you work - never let your patients know about these issues, and never let it interfere with the care you provide. Your patients are your priority; everything else is just background noise.

> 66 *Encountering this amount of politics at work was somewhat unexpected for me, and I'm starting to wonder whether everything generally is becoming more political, or whether I'm becoming less naive and only noticing it more now. To be honest I still don't really know, but I suspect it is the latter. There are times when I feel that everyone at work is feeling down because of these various political complaints and it is these moments where it is particularly difficult to stay upbeat. I try my absolute best to keep myself away from it all where possible, but it is hard not to get pulled into it. Just keep looking for the positives in every situation - change your outlook and you'll be happier; I've learnt that.* 99

Positivity is key; you can't change these situations, so why should you let them worry you?

Disagreements with colleagues

As explained in *Chapter Two*, working alongside doctors allows for a great relationship to be formed and makes patient care a lot easier. There might be times (although rare) where you find yourself disagreeing with a doctor over patient care, but you must remember at all times that you have to act in the best interest of your patient - you should never make a decision based on **your** beliefs and the doctor shouldn't do this based on **theirs**. The patient always, ALWAYS comes first. Sorry for the rant – see the personal account below for why this is so important to me.

> ❝ *I have only had a disagreement with a doctor on two occasions. The first instance was regarding a baby whose father was a friend of the consultant. He requested that the baby be discharged with an NG tube because she took 30 minutes to finish a bottle and the dad didn't want to 'waste his time' feeding her. The consultant then requested I pass the tube, but I refused to do so; the baby was feeding well (although slowly), was not getting tired and was gaining weight extremely well. I explained to the consultant the reasons why I didn't feel this was appropriate – the main one being that it wasn't in the patient's best interest. After a short battle of wills and a long chat with the father, he agreed with me and the baby went home tube-free.*
>
> *The second example was with regard to the patient I previously wrote about who refused to take her medication; I had been trying from 08.00 until 14.00 and she was point blank refusing it. When I explained this to the registrar and asked him to prescribe an alternative route his reply was 'you're not trying hard enough'. This comment really upset me because I had done absolutely everything I could think of, and he had seen her spit the medicine at me when we tried to hold her down. He later apologised for the way he spoke to me, but this is the most difficult situation I've ever had with a doctor. A difference of opinion is one thing, but being rude is another.* ❞

It can be very difficult to work alongside doctors if you disagree over the plan of care for your patient, but don't let this put you off questioning them. Having the confidence to do this comes with time, but you are well within your rights to refuse to do something if you firmly believe this will cause more harm than good. Below is a list of things to remember if you ever disagree with a doctor or medical professional.

» Regardless of whether you agree with their decision, you must respect them. Ask them to explain why they have chosen that course of treatment – they might have thought of something you hadn't, and if you still disagree, explain why.

» Becoming offensive or shouting will only cause the situation to escalate, and won't do anything to help your patient.

» Don't be afraid to question a doctor; if you don't understand how they've come to a decision, for example the calculation of a medication dose, query this with them. Going ahead might cause you to make a mistake.

» Go over their head – if a doctor is refusing to change their plan of care and you are certain that this is not in the best interests of your patient, don't be afraid to ask another doctor for their advice. The first doctor's ego might be bruised, but you will know that you're providing the best care possible for your patient.

Disagreements with your colleagues are never easy to deal with and can affect you for a long time, even after your shift has finished. If you are happy in the knowledge that your patient received the best care, then try not to dwell on an argument. If you can both move on, your working life will be so much easier – be civil if nothing else and you shouldn't have a problem.

Breaking bad news

Breaking bad news is never easy for anyone, and these situations are some of the hardest to be involved in. It's extremely rare that you'll be the one to break the news, as these things should always come from the doctors, but there is a chance you will be with the patient or relative when they are told. Your role in this will be to support your patient through whatever this news is, to help answer any questions they might have and to help them to come to terms with it. It is very important that this is done sensitively and with compassion in order to ensure the patient receives no additional emotional upset.

66 *Breaking bad news is never easy, and luckily it's not something I've often had to do. There is one instance that comes to my mind when thinking of this; I assisted a doctor who was informing a family that their child had leukaemia. This doctor is one of the most kind-hearted people I've ever been privileged to work with, and the way he informed the family of this news will stay with me forever; he was kind and compassionate in his words and he made the family feel so comforted. He allowed them time to come to terms with what they had been told,*

encouraged them to ask questions and didn't ever make them feel like they were eating into his time (even though he was meant to have finished his shift an hour previously - he didn't tell them that). It was only when the family went back to their room that he then became upset himself. 🙶

People's perceptions of what news is bad can be variable; one family will be very upset at something that another family will take in their stride, so be aware of this when informing them of any new diagnosis or change in their plan of care. For example, one family might be upset at the news of a chest infection, but another might be relieved that it is not something more sinister.

You're in the most caring profession, so I know that whichever way you approach this it will be handled with empathy and understanding. I can't tell you exactly what to do or say in these situations because each one is different and individual, but as long as you provide support and compassionate care to whoever needs it, you'll have done the best you can.

The death of a patient

This is never something that will be easy to deal with, no matter how often you do it. It's not something I've experienced very often *thankfully* so the advice I can offer here will be minimal. Instead this part will be told almost completely as personal accounts, and after each I will offer advice regarding what I have learned from each of these situations.

🙶 *My first experience of a patient's death was during my third year as a student nurse, on my A&E placement. A man who had had a cardiac arrest had been rushed into resus and although everything possible had been done, he was pronounced dead. They moved him into a side room for privacy, and once everything was ready the nurse asked if I would help her prepare his body to be taken to the mortuary. The nurse's care whilst doing this was truly remarkable - it obviously wasn't her first time but she still showed such respect and compassion. She explained to the man exactly what she was doing, she apologised to him because her hands were cold and she didn't try to make small talk with me. She remembered that this man was a person and treated him as such - it was really amazing and is something I will never forget.* 🙶

When our patients die it is important to remember that they are still people; whether they can hear us or know what we are doing, we must respect them. Although this aspect of caring for a deceased patient is hard, treating them in this way reminds us of our own humanity and the nurse's actions reassured me at this time that we don't get hardened to this, no matter how many times we experience it.

> **❝** My second experience was during my first winter as a qualified nurse. The patient was a baby with a life-limiting condition. He was admitted on our night shift, at the end of which I was discussing him with the day sister, saying that I was sure he would still be here this time next year. That night we came back into work and found out that he had passed away; that was hard. His family had left the ward already, so our support went to our team. The nurse in charge took it particularly hard; she stayed with us until 22.00 trying to ensure she had done absolutely everything she needed to, she phoned us at various points in tears and asking if she had missed anything, and then she came into work at 04.00 because she just wanted to be with us. It was so difficult to see our colleague this upset, but the way the team supported her through this was so touching and really highlighted to me the importance of teamwork. **❞**

The way a patient death affects the nursing team is very unique; some will touch us more than others and it can also depend on the level of input we've had. It is so important that we as a team support each other through these difficult times, but it can be hard to know how. In my experience, simply being there for them is enough; they will talk about it when they are ready and sometimes just having people around is all that they need.

> **❝** This account is slightly different; I was working on the children's ward, but an 18-month-old – Stacey (not her real name) – had been rushed into A&E. She was found collapsed in her bed and brought in by ambulance but despite the paramedic's attempts to revive her she was pronounced dead almost as soon as she arrived. Stacey had been an inpatient on our ward a few weeks earlier, so some of us knew the family already. During the middle of the morning we were informed that the girl's sister,

Cara, was to be admitted; Cara was generally unwell herself and they didn't know the cause of Stacey's death so to ensure there wasn't an underlying illness, the doctors wanted to admit Cara. This also provided a massive reassurance to her family. We allowed the family to come down to us in their own time, closed off a double-bedded bay for them and relaxed the visiting rules to ensure no one felt excluded. We supported the girls' parents by answering any questions they had, giving advice regarding Cara, providing tea and biscuits and just giving them time to come to terms with what had happened. They knew that we were there for them if they needed us, and we left them alone; they needed time together as a family, without the interference of even the most well-meaning of strangers/nurses. 🍣

This experience highlighted to me the importance of supporting the patient's family; whether expected or not, the death of a loved one will always be difficult to cope with, and people need time to come to terms with this. Offering support is extremely important, but so is giving them space and time to grieve. Most importantly, just be there for them when they need you.

The way we each deal with the death of our patient is different, and it can become a very emotional time for us as nurses. Some of us will cry with the family, others might cry secretly in a cupboard on the ward and some will be able to leave it behind. Although this can be a very difficult experience for us, it is important that we never let our own feelings overshadow those of our patient; crying with a family in supporting them is one thing, crying so much that they end up supporting us is another. Try to keep your patient and their family at the forefront of your mind, and take time for yourself later - if you feel that you really need to leave, then a colleague can step in while you regain composure.

When mistakes are made

Everyone's biggest worry when nursing is "What if I make a mistake?"; it's a completely normal concern and thankfully errors are rare. Mistakes come in all shapes and sizes but no matter what they are or whether we could have prevented them, they make us feel really awful. The main thing to remember at this point is that no one is going to hold it against you; mistakes are all about learning, not blaming. Most errors or mistakes do not require any further investigation once noticed and reported, but on the rare occasion that they do, please be assured that you will be properly supported through whatever may happen next.

If you do make a mistake, or notice that a mistake has been made, it is incredibly important that it is addressed and dealt with promptly by using the correct channels. For most (if not all) Trusts or healthcare providers the protocol is that you report it to:

» the nurse in charge – ensure the nurse in charge is made aware of the error as soon as it is recognised; they can then advise and support you regarding what happens next.

» the doctors – inform the doctors about any errors, particularly if this involves medication or a physical aspect of the patient's care. They will be able to assess the patient, establish if there is any harm or adverse effect and try to correct this if possible.

» the patient – if the mistake involves one particular patient, it is extremely important that they are made aware of what has happened and what might happen next. Apologising sincerely is the best way to go about this; if they can see you are genuinely sorry they are likely to be more forgiving. If the error was regarding medication then the patient should be closely monitored and informed of likely side-effects that they should look out for. You should also inform them of how to put in a complaint should they want to; this is not so that they can lay the blame on someone, but so that more measures can be put in place to stop this from re-occurring in the future. When telling a patient about an error it is advisable that you take someone else with you, just in case they become angry or volatile; it's also a good idea to have a second witness to the conversation.

» incident reporting software – any incident or near miss should be reported using your local reporting software, which for most of the UK is Datix. These reports are then sent to the relevant parties who can review the errors/near misses. Where required they can then investigate how they happened and the ways in which they can be prevented from happening in the future.

» the nurse who made the mistake (if this is not you) – they should also be made aware as soon as possible to ensure that they are properly supported through any investigation that follows. If you are the one to tell them, it is important to tell them somewhere private, not in front of their patients or colleagues, as this can put you both in a difficult situation. Discuss this sensitively as it is likely they are going to feel terrible, and remember that you are not laying the blame on them; mistakes can be made by anyone.

One very important thing to remember here is that no one is going to play the blame game. Accidents are just that: accidents. They aren't made on purpose; they happen, it's part of being human. Mistakes can be invaluable because they provide us with an opportunity for learning, particularly if they are small errors or near misses. Whatever might come next will depend on what it is that has happened:

>> You might require some extra training; for example, if the error involved medication you might have to complete a drug workbook or study day.

>> You might undergo a brief period of supervision until both you and your manager are happy that you are competent. An error is likely to knock your confidence so it might take time for you to feel comfortable with the particular skill.

>> Your manager might devise an addition protocol to ensure this does not happen in the future.

Whatever the outcome, your manager should ensure that you will receive any support you need; if you feel like you're on your own at any point speak to them.

If you have made an error, try not to dwell on it. As long as there is no lasting damage to a patient, you have reported it through the correct channels and it has been dealt with appropriately, there is nothing more you can do other than learn from it; anything else will only bring you down. If the mistake has been made by your colleague, your role will be to comfort them. They will be feeling terrible about what has happened and they will need a friend; always be that friend.

It is very important to note here that if you do make a mistake which has to be followed up, this will always be done confidentially between yourself and your manager; your colleagues will never be informed of anything that will happen regarding further investigations unless you tell them yourself (and you don't need to tell them anything you don't want them to know).

Shortly after I had revalidated I attended a study day where we were taught about the concepts of 'Human Factors' and 'Black Box Thinking' - an integral aspect within the aviation industry. Linking this to the NHS is airline pilot Martin Bromiley, whose wife Elaine tragically died following routine surgery when her airway collapsed during the anaesthetic process. As a pilot Bromiley stated that he is aware of the important checks that are carried out before any flight and the way any incidents are investigated. He quickly realised how differently the NHS could deal with mistakes if this stance was adopted - any error, no matter how tragic, can be learned from. I won't go into this too deeply, but I would definitely recommend that you look into this story - put Martin or Elaine's name into any search engine and you will find out the information. The take-home message from this is that trying to lay blame on someone won't get you anywhere, but reflecting on and learning from mistakes can make a massive difference to the way you work and to your patients in the future; this is so important.

How to cope with difficult situations

It's important to recognise that along the way you will come across some situations that you might find difficult. I felt these important to write about because they are all things that I've struggled with and for me it would have been good to know that other people feel this way too; that's my aim for this whole book.

If you can relate to any of the topics I've written about in this chapter, you'll know how important it is to be able to move on from them. If you're struggling with this, there are a few tips that I hope you find helpful at the end of the next chapter - feel free to flick forward and have a look. I find it useful to: reflect, talk to someone, have a little cry if I need to, stay busy until I can properly take time and focus on the positives.

TOP TIPS

★ Patients will quite often cause us some emotional distress, and if this does happen you're allowed time to be upset. Try to ensure that your patient doesn't see this, though, and remember that they are your priority first and foremost.

★ Patients who are aggressive or uncooperative can also be very difficult to deal with. Always remember that there might be a legitimate reason for their frustration and try to understand this when talking to them. Never let yourself become vulnerable, however, and if you feel as if a situation is escalating then it's best to take yourself out of it and get help.

★ Politics is a big thing within nursing and you're never going to get away from it. Although it's a lot easier said than done, try not to let yourself get too involved in it, and try not to let it get you down; if you can't change it, why should you let it get to you?

★ The death of a patient will always be one of the most difficult things you will have to deal with as a nurse. In these situations it is vital that you always treat the patient and their family with utmost respect and allow them their own time to come to terms with what has happened. Be a source of support for your patient, their family and your colleagues, and remember that you are allowed to cry - you're human after all.

★ Making a mistake is a big fear for every nurse, but if this does happen to you the most important thing to remember is that you should always be honest about what has happened. You will receive the support you need and everything that happens will remain confidential. Get into the habit of taking away the blame and learning from mistakes; this will allow for better patient care in the future and a more positive outlook for you and your colleagues.

GOOD DAYS AND BAD DAYS

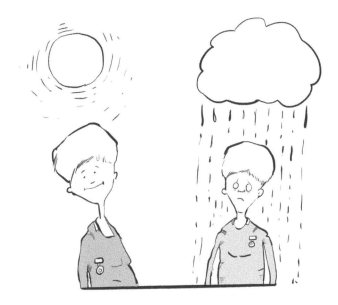

It's rare that we remember the really good days, unless a certain patient or event has made it memorable. My aim for this chapter is to help you (and me) remember the really wonderful things about nursing - the reasons we entered this vocation, and the reasons we stay in it.

However, when bad days happen they can really knock your confidence, so this chapter will also explore why this is, how you can avoid it and how to turn a bad day into a good one. To close the chapter I have included a section about how to help yourself recover from a bad day; this is something that I believe to be very important for every nurse - you need to look after yourself as well as your patients.

N.B. I refer to 'days' a lot here, but this of course applies to whatever different shifts we work.

Good days

Most of our days at work will be good ones and will be the reason that we love nursing so much. We nurses have an innate ability to see the good in almost every situation; there is something about it that just makes us happy, and I can't quite put my finger on what it is. There are times when we can have the busiest of days, but still come away from work feeling extremely happy; it's a very strange feeling. I was recently reminded of something I'd posted on a certain social media site when I was in my second year of university (five years ago – how time flies!):

> 66 *I'm sure it's not natural to walk out of an extremely busy 12½ hour shift and feel this amazingly happy! Good career choice? I DEFINITELY think so!* 99

It's really great to be able to look back at posts such as these and be reminded that this wonderful career has been so rewarding from the very beginning. Despite frequently having extremely busy shifts, if we know we have helped someone in some small way, then we can come away having had a great day. I think that's what nursing is all about; we help make a difference in people's lives, and that's a wonderful thing to be able to do.

> 66 *It's so common that I will reach the end of a shift and have a sudden adrenaline rush. Is this because I'm finally free? Possibly, but I think it's more to do with the fact that I've had a really great day. When I know I've done the absolute best that I can for my patients I'm always happy, but when I know I've gone above and beyond for them, I'm usually dancing out of work and high-fiving myself! These are the best days – and they are so common; I must remember this!* 99

What makes our shifts good?

Most days at work are good ones, even if they are busy. There are several reasons that this is the case, such as:

» Great patients – as explained in *Chapter Three*, we have the opportunity to build up a great relationship with our patients, and we spend most of our day with them. They are usually the determining factor as to whether we have a good day or a bad one. Sometimes, this can be the patients themselves, and sometimes it's the situation involving our patients, for example:

> › Knowing that we have made a difference in the lives of our patients is a really wonderful feeling, and it's probably the one we get most often. Sometimes our patients will personally thank us

for our help and care, other times we will see a difference in them and know that we have helped.

> If our patients are friendly and we can build a good relationship with them it will be extremely difficult to come away feeling that we have had a hard day. Working cooperatively alongside our patients allows everything to run smoothly and will help us to give them the best possible care. If we can have a chat or a laugh with them at the same time, that's even better! Patients like these will always impact us in a very positive way, and they really make the job worthwhile.

> Getting positive feedback from patients and relatives is a really wonderful way to help remind us what a great job we do, and it's lovely for our hard work to be noticed. This positive feedback can make a bad day 100 times better and reminds us why we are in this profession; we can make a difference.

66 It's always a joy to care for families who are truly lovely people and are grateful for anything you can do for them. This can really turn a bad day into a good one, something that I was reminded of very recently. I had worked a night shift where we admitted a baby who had to be kept nil by mouth (which I'm sure you'll agree is difficult for a baby). Poor mum was completely exhausted, and we noticed that the baby was becoming very unsettled because he could smell mum's milk. I offered to put him in his pram and go for a walk to settle him to sleep, so mum could also get some rest. This worked almost instantly, and he then slept for the whole night (and importantly, so did mum). A few days later I was on a day shift and I was assigned to look after the baby again. This shift was a busy one and I found myself struggling to stay positive at times. When the baby was discharged his mum gave me a box of biscuits to say thank you because she was so grateful for my help on the previous shift. I was so touched by this and it really reminded me that although we have hard days, I really do love my job; I made a difference to my patient and his family, and they were grateful for it. That's the best feeling ever. 99

» Great staffing - any shift you're working with a team who are just that - a team - is going to be a good one, regardless of what the ward is like at the time. I mentioned this back in *Chapter Two*, and I firmly believe that if there is a great team on (and you have the right amount of staff), you're almost guaranteed to have a good day. Knowing that no matter what happens there's always someone who can help is a great reassurance, and if you get those rare times where you can sit and have a laugh with your colleagues it really lifts your spirits. At the end of the shift you can party out of the doors together knowing you've all done an amazing job!

> 66 *There have been so many instances where we have had a really good day because of the team we've been working with. Even if it has been incredibly busy or there has been a heavy workload, having the help of brilliant colleagues is priceless and when we all stay positive we really lift each other up. We always joke that we are 'The A Team' or 'The Dream Team', and most days that is so true; it's great to work with your friends!* 99

» A great outlook - always believe in the power of positive thought. I'm sure you'll recognise that I've said this a lot throughout this book, but I really do think it works. If you're sceptical about this, let me expand: if you can start your shift thinking "It's going to be a good day" and maintain this outlook, it will take a lot to stop you having a good day. It's important to try to see the good in every situation - if you can do this, then your whole outlook will improve. Although this is difficult, I would definitely recommend that you give it a try. Have a look at the flow chart below for my own simple (but maybe too simplistic?!) way of dealing with this; then look a little lower for some real advice:

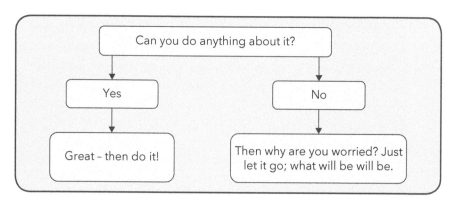

On a serious note, if I'm in a tricky situation I usually ask myself one of two questions:

1) Is there anything you can do to change what has happened/will happen? The answer to this is usually no, so if there is nothing you can do about it, why worry? Just do what you can do, and that will be more than enough.

2) Will you still be affected by this in a year's time? A university lecturer once asked us this question, and I've always remembered it; if it won't affect you a week, a month or a year from now, then why worry about it? Worrying only makes the situation seem much worse, but if you can disregard it and move on you'll feel much better about it.

There might be some instances where these won't apply, but on the whole, most causes for worry at work will fall into one of these two categories; I've yet to come across one that doesn't. If you really feel like you're struggling to stay positive though, please do speak to your manager or someone you trust about this; don't suffer in silence.

» When things run smoothly – the most satisfying kinds of days are those when everything goes exactly to plan: all of your observations are performed on time, your patients are lovely and extremely compliant with absolutely everything that you need to do, the doctor's round finishes promptly and the discharges are ready when you need them, all of your IVs are given perfectly with no cannulas tissuing and you are up to date with your notes by the time handover rolls around. This might sound like a fairytale or the plot for the latest Disney film, but there are occasions when it does happen, and it feels really great! There have been many instances when things have gone exactly to plan, but there have also been many instances where they haven't. Although it is a wonderful feeling to be able to do absolutely everything when it is required, don't write it off if it doesn't happen:

    ❝ *There have been several occasions where nothing has happened at the right time, but everything still works out fine. This is largely due to having understanding and trusting patients/parents. I still vividly remember one parent in particular whose child had been on our ward for almost a month and today was the day she was finally going to be discharged. The discharge letter was completed, the TTOs had been delivered and as soon as the final dose of IV antibiotic was given they would be allowed to go home. On this occasion (as it always seems to be) the child's cannula tissued as we were flushing prior to giving the dose. Typical to occasions such as this, the doctors had been called to an emergency in A&E and there was no one on the ward who could cannulate. Instead of moaning and complaining like a lot of people would have done, this mum laughed, shrugged and said 'not to worry - we were the emergency in A&E last month so let them take their time'. This outlook from a parent is exactly the sort we all need in times like this - she was happy to wait until someone was available and didn't make a fuss or try to complain about the situation. The doctors were back from the emergency within around an hour, they successfully cannulated her and the IV was given. The patient was discharged home and we haven't seen her since - that was a very good day.* 🙶

What do you think?

I recently asked some student nurses via social media about how we know we've had a good day, and I was delighted to read so many wonderful responses. The majority of us agree that it's mostly down to our patients; if we know we have made a difference to at least one person then it has been a good day. Another common theme was being made to feel part of the nursing team, regardless of whether we are new or 'temporary'.

Those who contributed their experiences are happy for me to include them in this chapter, and I'm so pleased to be sharing them with you now:

Marie said:

"As an LD student a positive interaction makes my day. I recently worked with a man who had never spoken a word for so long it was thought that he was non-verbal. Within three shifts with him he said his first word to me. This was possibly the best moment of my training so far and I have just finished my second year."

Poppy said:
"Being able to form a relationship with my patients. I'm in theatres at the moment which means you have to build this quick and gain trust. I love making my patients smile."

Lauren said:
"When the person you're looking after is smiling and thanking you for everything you've done for them. Makes everything worthwhile and can easily turn a hectic/bad day into a really positive one."

Rachel said:
"When your patients give you feedback. I have had patients literally grab my hand as I go past and tell me they have seen I am a caring/compassionate person, which I strive to be, so I am thrilled it comes across that way to patients. Also reminds me to always be on my game, as our lovely patients often have very little to do but sit by their beds and watch the staff around them (of course depending on the ward/client group). Also, seeing patients smile! Especially those who have been understandably distressed and upset, to see them smile makes my day – and when I tell them so, they smile even more!

Being included in the team, despite only being there temporarily; you can always tell which nurses remember what it is like to be a student/new to a team, and it makes such a difference to be included.

Practically, when I achieve something I have been afraid of, e.g. handing over the entire ward to the whole team; my mentor told me from day one that would be a goal she would set for me, and I was so afraid, but having done it, I was proud of myself and really enjoyed it. Will ask to do it again on my next shift!"

Naomi said:
"The two biggest things that put a smile on my face are:

1. When I successfully undertake skills that I've struggled with in the past, no matter how small (put a Conveen on for the first

time the other day, stupidly proud of myself) and
2. The service users and their families; I love the personal interactions, the give and take of trust and vulnerability. I love when the connection finally clicks into place and you know that they value you and the care you provide. That moment is what keeps me getting up at 5am and going back every day."

Jasmine said:
"I'm currently looking after a young man who's been hospitalised for three months so far. His mental health is bad and in the three months he's been with us (I'm currently on a respiratory ward for placement) he's learnt to talk, eat, walk and gain independence again. Myself and my mentor are fighting to get him funding to get a supportive living home. Today he said how well I've developed as a nurse and how I've inspired him to become a support worker or even a nurse one day from reflecting from my work.
MY EYES WELLED UP."

I am so grateful for the comments I received regarding this, and it is really wonderful to be able to connect with other nurses and students and be reminded exactly why we are all in this job - most importantly, it's about the patients. Your comments (and don't stop them coming, I'd love to hear more about why people have had good days - have a look at the *Me and My Book* section at the beginning of the book for ways to connect with me) can really help inspire and encourage others, particularly if they are struggling to see the light at the end of the tunnel. We nurses have to stick together; we help each other celebrate the good times and console each other through the difficult times.

Bad days

Bad days are generally few and far between, but if you have a number of them in quick succession they can get on top of you, and it can sometimes feel like you're never going to get over this cycle. This is something I have struggled with a lot, and a lot of my friends who are newly qualified have too. If you can finish a shift and know you've given your patient the best care that you possibly can, then you've done a good job.

Firstly, let me reassure you that it will get better – bad days don't last forever and as you grow in confidence you will find your own ways to deal with them. I definitely had my share of days when I started where I didn't know if I was coming or going, but along the way I've learned ways to manage my workload and overcome some of these problems. Don't get me wrong, I still have bad days, but I deal with them much better now. I'll explore some of the ways I have done this a little bit later in the chapter, so sit tight.

Why do bad days happen?

The answers to this question are mostly the reverse of the previous section. There are many factors that contribute to bad days, such as a heavy patient workload or poor staffing levels or skill mix. A busy day doesn't always mean a bad day, but there is a fine line between 'busy' and 'too busy', and when that line is crossed it becomes very difficult. There are three main reasons that we might have a bad day:

» Poor staffing levels or skill mix – when you're not fully staffed the workload instantly increases and this can put extra strain on you and your colleagues. Similarly, if the skill mix is poor your workload might increase; this will become more prominent to you as you progress in your career.

» Heavy patient workload – having a lot of patients doesn't always equate to a busy shift if they are straightforward ones, but when there is a lot to be done or things don't go to plan, this can instantly increase your workload and might mean that you have less time to spend with them or other patients.

» Poor expectation of your shift – as explained above, if you have a lot of bad days in quick succession, it can change the way you feel about work; if you're expecting a shift to go badly, the likelihood is that it will. Don't feel bad if you think this way; it's human nature and we are all entitled to our 'down days'. Sometimes things that are happening outside of work can impact the way we feel inside work. I will expand on this further in *Chapter Seven: Work/life balance*.

    66 Looking back on the bad days I have had, there always seems to be one common thread; when 'busy' becomes 'too busy'. I'm a bit of a stress-head and if I start to lose control of what's going on, I begin to get flustered. I find that organisation is extremely important in managing a heavy workload and I am getting better at that as time goes by (but I do still have a lot of room for improvement in this area). My main worry, however, is when it becomes unsafe; I've had too many shifts where I find myself unable to do any more than the absolute basics of what is required of me and it really scares me. What if I make a mistake? What if I miss something? What if my patient is really sick and I've been too busy to notice? These days are, of course, massively outweighed by days where I don't have this worry, but at the time it can be really scary. 🙶

How to help yourself have a good day

» Poor staffing or skill mix? As you progress you might find that you're helping your more junior colleagues (which of course is absolutely fine and no one would ever refuse to help) – it's a great way to help them learn and 'pass the baton' but it can mean that the extra workload makes your shift busier. I always try my absolute utmost to help other members of my team, whether they are junior or senior to me, but I do find that sometimes I need to ask them to do something in return. In *Chapter One* I wrote about this in reverse; if someone helps you with something, think about what you can do for them. When you're in the opposite situation, don't be afraid to ask them to do something for you; it will help them to gain expertise in this task, and really helps them to feel an important member of your nursing team. Teamwork is about sharing workload and that's the best way to manage a busy ward.

» Heavy patient workload – this is something that isn't necessarily going to be easy to get around, as a heavy workload is one of the most difficult aspects of this job. I find that organisation is the key; one of my colleagues (a genius) created a 'time sheet' so that we could write down which patient needs what interventions every hour, and they have become very effective for most people – it becomes easy to keep track of your patients and ensure nothing gets missed. However, I (awkward as usual) find that on an average day I will fill this sheet in first thing, but from 10 o'clock onwards I don't take it out of my pocket. The times I do find it extremely helpful are when I have a heavier workload and therefore things need to be done on time. There will be days where you can't get everything done that you need to, and you'll have to hand jobs over to the next shift; that's just how it goes, and that's fine.

> 66 It can be hard to put a positive spin on a busy day; and you can very quickly feel deflated if you don't feel you've done enough for your patients; however, my outlook is: if I have done everything required of me by the end of the shift and my patients are better (or at least no worse) than when I started, I consider this to be a job well done. Of course, it's wonderful to be able to go the extra mile for our patients and on days where this is possible it's really brilliant, but when it has been busy or I have a heavy workload I've learned to be content in the knowledge that I have done all I can for my patients, and have helped them. Some days that has to be enough, but it has taken me three years to begin to realise this. 99

Below is a template of the time sheet used by many of my colleagues (and myself on special occasions):

	08:00	09:00	10:00	11:00	12:00	13:00	14:00	15:00	16:00	17:00	18:00	19:00
Bed 1												
Bed 2												
Bed 3												
Bed 4												
Bed 5												

» Poor expectation of the shift – I covered this to an extent in the above section regarding good days, but one more thing I would like to share with you here is this: when I first qualified I found that I was having as many bad days as good ones, but I soon realised that if I wrote down what had made my days good, I could look back over them after a bad day and remind myself that I really do love my job, so that's what I did. I find this very beneficial, not only because it allows me to look back at the list when I'm struggling, but also, finishing a shift and highlighting what was good about it helps me look for the positives in every situation. If you do this after every bad day they will quickly become good days in your mind – the power of positive thought! That is something I would always recommend people do, as we sometimes do need reminding of how amazing our vocation can be. Another way to do this is to save comments or cards/gifts from patients. This is useful both for revalidation (see *Chapter Eight*) and to remind us of the difference that we are making every day.

Excerpts from my list of positives (I've changed the dates to protect confidentiality):

> *12th September 2016: "Today was busy and I didn't really get a chance to stop, but I assisted a doctor with an LP [lumbar puncture] which came back negative thankfully, but also as a 'champagne tap' – the consultant told me this is where there are no red blood cells; a perfect LP. He shook my hand and said 'It's all down to the holding – back in the day I'd have bought you a bottle of champagne!' I felt weirdly proud – but unfortunately I never did get that bottle!"*
>
> *8th November 2016: "We had an amazing team on today and all of my patients were such lovely people. I spent about half an hour chatting to one mum about her kids (who are hilarious! I need to meet them all!)."*
>
> *1st January 2017: "Busy busy busy day today – it was hard to stay positive. My patient ended up getting retrieved (transferred to a specialist hospital in London) because he has meningococcal septicaemia. Luckily it was recognised quickly and it was more of an elective transfer than emergency, but his poor family are so stressed. As they were leaving I wished the family well and said that I hoped we would see him back with us soon. His Nan put her hand on my arm and said 'I can see this is hard for you, but you're a wonderful nurse. Thank you.' It took everything I had not to cry at that point, but it really showed me that I am making a difference."*

Sick patients

On some shifts you might have fewer, more unwell patients to care for. Some people prefer this as they can focus all of their care on one person; others prefer to have lots of different things to do rather than focus on one person in particular. There will come a time when you will be allocated to care for these patients, and if you haven't often done this it can be scary and quite demanding. The first few times you care for these patients you might come away thinking you've had a really bad day but the more you do it, the more confident you'll become; it's good to get used to it. The next chapter will explore this more fully in terms of growing in confidence and caring for sicker patients, but for now I will focus on those times when your patient unexpectedly becomes unwell.

When our patients suddenly take a turn for the worse whilst in our care, it can become really terrifying. We can get swept up in the urgency that ensues (we alert everyone that we need to and assist in ensuring that they get the correct treatment promptly) and sometimes it doesn't fully hit us until the event has ended. It is then that we might feel awful about it; perhaps our concern is that they aren't going to get better or we worry that we didn't recognise something soon enough. This can be hard to move on from, but talking to someone with experience about this will definitely help you to feel reassured.

> 66 The first time this happened to me was really terrifying; I was looking after a one-year-old girl who had a chest infection. I was doing her observations half hourly and they had been stable so I discussed this with the nurse in charge and we decided that they could be done hourly. I then took this opportunity to go on my break but was halfway through when the nurse in charge came in and told me that the little girl had developed severe increased work of breathing and almost had a respiratory arrest. She requested that I go up to theatres with the patient and the doctors as she needed to be intubated and transferred out. This whole event remains a complete blur to me and I was just focusing on making sure that everything the theatre staff requested was done. In total it took an hour and a half for her to be retrieved, and it was only when I returned to the ward that it really hit me: did I miss something? Was I wrong to extend the frequency of her obs? I felt really awful about this so I asked the SHO and nurse in charge what had happened and if there was anything I could have done. They took me aside and fully explained to me exactly what had happened and that there was absolutely nothing more I could have done; children are unpredictable and go downhill quickly. I felt so reassured about this after talking to them, and within a few days the patient was transferred back to us, almost completely recovered. 99

If you're in this situation, the main thing to remember is that there is no shame in asking for help. If you feel like you aren't coping with your patients, speak to the nurse in charge; they might be able to help you or to reallocate so that you don't have as many patients. It's always good to have experience in caring for sicker patients, but you need to feel ready for this. You might get swept up in the situation, so when it's over it can be really helpful to talk it through with someone more senior, whether this be a nurse or doctor. They can explain exactly what happened and why it happened, and this knowledge will help you if the situation ever occurs again.

How to recover from a bad day

Recovering from a bad day is so important; you need to be able to move on from the events in order to avoid 'burning out', a concept which will be explored more deeply in *Chapter Seven*. There are many ways in which you can recover from a bad day; sometimes this will happen unexpectedly whilst you're still at work, other times it will require something specific such as making a conscious effort to relax or reflect following a hard shift. The more bad days you have, the better you will become at recovering from them, but it might take you a little time to find the best way to do this. I have learned that after a bad day a cup of tea (you might prefer a glass of wine), a bath, sometimes a little cry (because there is absolutely nothing wrong with letting it out) and an early night normally sort me out and I can *usually* wake up the next day feeling better and ready to start all over again.

> 66 *Generally if I am having a bad day at work I expect it to remain bad until the end of my shift, but on some occasions something can happen that will magically make everything better. My favourite time this has ever happened was a few months after my revalidation when we had a baby on the ward who had been there for three months and whose parents were unable to stay with her for very long. This meant that the nursing and play team could spend time with her when she was alone (and when we got the chance) and so we got to know her very well. One day I found myself having a hard time so I went in to see how our little baby was doing. I was chatting and playing with her when all of a sudden she gave me a big smile and started to laugh. That was the first time I had ever heard her*

do this, and in that second it just made everything OK. Little moments like this are so special, and I really cherish them. **„**

Some days we might have to make a conscious effort to make ourselves feel better, and there are many ways in which this can be done. This aspect also applies to the previous chapter, as difficult situations and bad days can be much the same thing. The advice is as follows:

» Relaxation - for me, this is the best way to get over a difficult day. I get home from work, run a hot bath, make a cup of tea and dig out a good book. This instantly helps to take my mind off whatever has happened and allows me to relax and prepare for an early night - particularly helpful if I'm back in work the following day.

» Written reflection - this is an extremely useful way to deal with any bad day or emotional difficulty, and you can do this in a variety of ways. Writing things down is a very good way to get your emotions out there and help you deal with them. This will also come in handy for your revalidation - see *Chapter Eight*.

» Talk about it - another way of reflecting (which we almost always do without giving it a second thought) is through talking. We talk to our colleagues, our families, our pets and sometimes ourselves. We speak about what happened and how it affected us, and this helps us to deal with what we are experiencing. Most (if not all) occupational health departments will offer some kind of counselling service, so if you feel you need it, have a chat with them. Whichever way you reflect on the day's events, it's important that you do reflect; bottling things up will only weigh you down.

» There's nothing wrong with a good cry - some people deal with difficult situations by bursting into tears. This can be because you feel frustrated, upset or just because you've become overwhelmed with the situation. There is absolutely nothing wrong with this; crying can be very therapeutic. My only advice here would be that you ensure this doesn't interfere with your patient care, and that you try to take yourself away - patients don't need to see their nurse getting upset.

» Keep yourself busy - this is almost the opposite of the above point, but this is how some people cope with difficult situations. Keeping busy will help to keep your mind off what has happened, but remember to look after yourself. This response will usually end in one of two ways; either you will get to the end of the shift and almost have forgotten about the situation, or you'll finish your shift, relax and it will hit you. Whichever way you deal with this might be fine for you, but if you're the latter kind of person it's extremely important that you don't let it affect you for too long after your shift has ended. I recently read a book by comedian Sarah Millican who gave some really great advice; she calls it 'Millican's Law' and although she is referring to her comedy, I really liked it and found it applicable to nursing. It goes like this (I'll paraphrase): if you've had a hard day, you're only allowed to feel down about it until 11am (or pm if you're on nights) the next day; by this point you should be able to put it all behind you and move on. I would personally change the time slightly to whenever you wake up the next day as being sad until 11 o'clock can be tricky if you're back in work, but I really love the principle. If you do find yourself becoming pulled down by what is happening at work, talk to someone.

» Focus on the positive - in every difficult situation there will be a little glimmer of happiness; find it and focus on it. Think about how you made your patient smile; how you made the end of their life as peaceful as possible; how you ensured your patient received the correct dose when you questioned the prescription; how your support helped a family who have just lost a relative. Maintaining a positive outlook goes a long way towards helping you to cope with these situations, no matter how difficult.

I will leave you with a reminder that **you are an amazing nurse**. Bad days are inevitable and sometimes are more frequent than we would like, but a bad day doesn't mean a bad job. If you are struggling please talk to someone; whether this is a family member, your line manager, a fellow colleague, anyone - don't bottle it up and let it get you down. Focus on the good times and they will get you through the bad; you're doing a really great job.

TOP TIPS

★ We all have good days and we all have bad days. Take each shift as it comes and let them mould you into the fantastic nurse that you are.

★ It's really important to enjoy good days when they come – they are brilliant in reminding us why we do the job that we do, and they're so common!

★ Our patients are the primary reason that we have good days; knowing that we have helped someone and made a difference in their lives is the best feeling, and when we see the change that we are making, we feel like superheroes (which we are!).

★ Bad days might feel very frequent at times, but try not to let them get you down. This is a lot easier said than done, I know, but try to take time after each shift to look for the positives, even if there is only one. Getting into this habit can really help to change your outlook on your working life, and might just help you to recover from these bad shifts when they occur.

★ Always talk to someone if you are struggling with work. This doesn't have to be someone at work, it can be anyone; just don't bottle everything up because at some point you'll just go bang. Please look after yourself and remember how amazing you are!

PROGRESSION AND CONFIDENCE

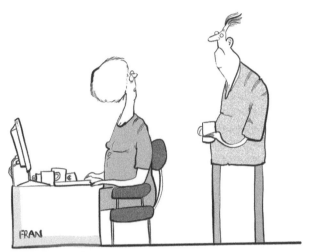

I can fit in all my study days as long as I work a nine day week.

As your first three years as a qualified nurse progress, your confidence will also build. This chapter will explore this, looking into the ways that we progress and highlighting how to know when we are ready. Starting from your preceptorship period and working towards progressing higher up the bands, this chapter will discuss the ways in which we develop as nurses; both through study days and through learning on the job. I will also explore the ways in which caring for high dependency patients can affect our confidence and how we might know when we are ready to start taking these patients (usually through being thrown in at the deep end!). Becoming a mentor is also an aspect of progression and working alongside students can do wonders for your confidence, so this will also be explored later in the chapter.

Preceptorship period

I covered this topic in *Chapter One* so I won't spend too much time on it here, but as previously mentioned, when you first qualify you will have an initial period of preceptorship. This is recommended by the NMC and should be an official agreement between you and your manager. You'll be allocated a 'preceptor' who can help support and guide you during this time and you might be given some workbooks to complete, such as medicines management or competencies for skills relating to your field of work. You should have regular meetings with your preceptor to address any learning needs or issues you might have and they can help to ensure you're appropriately supported through these. Every workplace runs differently, but if you aren't offered this experience you should talk to your manager and agree on a programme that suits you both.

Although most preceptorship programmes officially last for six months, in reality you will be consolidating your learning for any time between six months and three years; everyone works at their own pace. Don't worry if you don't feel ready – that will come with confidence.

> 66 When I was around eight or nine months qualified I was talking to a colleague about preceptorship who stated that although officially this ends at six months, she feels that you're not fully consolidated until you've been qualified for around two years. At the time I strongly agreed with her; two years seemed like an important milestone, by which time I'd have a lot more confidence and be fully comfortable in my role. When I reached this two-year mark, however, I suddenly felt very differently about this – I didn't feel that anything had really changed and I certainly didn't feel that I had 100% consolidated all of my knowledge. I still don't feel like I have and now I'm three and a half years qualified. 99

Confidence

Confidence is a big thing within nursing, and you will find that the longer you're working, the more confident you'll become. Some people start work with a great amount of confidence; they can get into the swing of it very quickly and you'd never know they are new. Others (including me) take a lot longer to come out of their shell and properly settle into their role. This doesn't mean that the latter are not as competent as the former, it simply means that we doubt ourselves more and maybe worry more. This isn't a bad thing; but it might mean that at the very beginning it's harder; bad days will seem much worse and good days will offer little consolation for this.

Confidence is a funny old thing; you can lose it as quickly as you gain it, and vice versa. You might start a shift feeling like SuperNurse, but something can happen that will knock you back and you'll spend the rest of the shift trying to claw back any kind of faith you had in yourself. I find that the amount of confidence I have varies from shift to shift and depends on a variety of different factors, as I'm sure it does for most people. These factors might be:

» Patient load - if I have a lot of patients, or patients who are particularly unwell, my confidence might drop a little until I am sure that they are stable and that the care I'm giving them is working.

» Skill mix - this one is more psychological, I think, but I find that the more senior support I have, the more I feel like I need it. For example, if I am one of the most junior on the shift, I have less confidence because I know my colleagues are there if I need them - it doesn't make much sense, but maybe it's the security of knowing they're there.

» Recent events - if something has happened recently that has knocked my confidence, it can take a while for this to build back up; even if it was something small.

&& *My third winter of working was particularly busy, and I remember one shift I was caring for a patient who had a lower respiratory tract infection. This patient was on humidified high flow oxygen and was coping with this very well; however, at 05.00 he began to deteriorate; his saturations were dropping despite me increasing his oxygen and he was extremely unsettled. Between the hours of 05.00 and 07.00 I was in his cubicle constantly, trying everything I could think of to help bring his sats up, but nothing seemed to be working. I asked the nurse in charge for help, but she couldn't think of any other ways to help him that I hadn't already tried. The longer this went on for, the worse it seemed, and when the day staff came around I felt ashamed to be telling them that I just didn't know what else to do. They (of course) were extremely understanding and reassured me that they would try to fix him during the day (which they did because they are superstars!) but I still cried on the way home. When I returned that night and was allocated a different patient with the same respiratory condition, I suddenly felt like I could no longer trust my instinct and was relying on my senior colleagues for advice about everything. I don't know why at that time I felt so out of my depth – normally I have no problems with caring for respiratory patients; it's 90% of our ward in the winter months – but sometimes it really does creep up on me.* **"**

Being confident in your job is the best feeling in the world – you feel like there is nothing you can't handle; all of your patients have received the best care they possibly can and you're having an amazing day. If you think back to your shifts recently, I'm sure you can pinpoint the times when you felt like this, and (almost certainly) that's the majority of the time.

If, like me, you feel like you're lacking in confidence, please let me reassure you that it does come with time, even if you have setbacks along the way. If you're looking to improve this, there are many ways in which it can be done:

» Experience – the more experience you have in your job, or in a particular aspect of your job, the more confident you will become.

» Knowledge – with knowledge comes confidence. This might be a bold statement to make, but I really believe this to be true (at least most of the time). If you have knowledge about something in particular, whether this be a system within the body or a piece of equipment used in your field, then having that knowledge and applying it to practice will have a monumental effect on your confidence as a nurse, particularly when you see the positive effect it has on your patient(s).

» Skill – the more skills you have under your belt, the more faith you'll have in yourself as a nurse. The ability to put these skills into practice is a great way to help build your confidence, especially when you do it often or if it's something you've struggled with in the past.

» Teaching – as you progress you might start to mentor students, work with newly qualified nurses or be able to share your experience with others in your team. Passing on your knowledge and skills is a great way to help you acknowledge just how much you know; even if this is the first time you realise it.

Study days

Study days are an important part of nursing and are extremely beneficial ways to expand your knowledge and develop your confidence, and any study day can be used for your revalidation portfolio. Nursing is ever-changing, so there will always be scope to learn something new that will help you to develop your skills and knowledge within your field – it's really exciting!

Mandatory study days (such as moving and handling, fire safety or conflict resolution) are vital in ensuring that you are able to practise safely in accordance with the policies and procedures in your place of work. Non-mandatory training is of equal importance; this applies to any training that is more in-depth and specific, and which will help you to develop knowledge and skills within your particular field of nursing.

> 66 When I had been qualified for around a year we had a lot of newly qualified nurses starting so our manager trialled a 'rolling programme' of training for us. This consisted of one study day a month, each on a different topic that will help expand our knowledge and improve our skills regarding the most common illnesses and conditions we are likely to see. This was extremely successful and has continued since then, now being offered to all nurses, not just those newly qualified. The impact this had for me on my knowledge and confidence was brilliant, and I feel that I have benefited greatly from these opportunities for learning. 99

Although they are most vital when you're newly qualified, it is important to continue to keep up to date and further your knowledge throughout your whole career. Without realising it you'll be learning and adapting your practice as you progress, but as nursing is always subject to change, keeping on top of the newest research and advancements in your field is the best way to ensure that you provide your patients with the highest standard of care possible. Attending study days is just one way that you can do this, but you can also stay up to date by:

» Reading the most recent articles, research and publications – this can be both online or in journals.

» Taking part in online discussions – there are many ways that you can do this; for example, the Twitter community: @wenurses hold weekly discussions on their Twitter feed and encourage nurses from everywhere to take part and share their experiences, thoughts and opinions.

» Taking part in online courses – a lot of websites for medical conditions offer free education on their websites that will help you to stay on top of the most recent advances in research. A great example of this is the UK Sepsis Trust website www.sepsistrust.org (although there are loads and loads of others, so have a look) which offers several online courses and educational resources for both health professionals and members of the public.

» Researching specific conditions or treatments – this is something we do without even thinking about it; if there is a condition that I haven't heard of or don't know much about, a little internet search will provide me with loads of information surrounding it. I can then pass this on to patients and their families to ensure they are provided with the most accurate information related to their admission. The NHS Choices website (www.nhs.uk) is great for this as it gives non-biased information in simple terms regarding a wide range of conditions.

As well as expanding your knowledge, learning new skills is also an important part of nursing. You'll have been doing this since you began your training, and there will always be more skills to learn along the way. Once you're properly settled into your role, you'll probably be put onto the intravenous administration course. Different work settings will offer this at different times – for me it was offered after six months, once I had completed my preceptorship booklet. The ability to do IVs is a big step towards autonomy, and for me, it was then that I felt like I could stop bothering my colleagues and do my work myself (although they never saw it like that).

There will always be skills that you will learn to help you as you progress in your career, and these will mostly be related to your speciality. For example, if you work on a busy ward you might learn skills in phlebotomy and cannulation; if you're a community district nurse you will learn additional skills in changing dressings and wound healing; if you're a mental health nurse you'll learn further conflict resolution, for example. Some of these will be learned in a study day setting, but most will be picked up while you're at work.

Learning 'on the job'

Although study days are extremely valuable ways to help us expand our knowledge, most of our learning takes place 'on the job'. From practising new skills to sharing thoughts and ideas with our colleagues, not a day goes by where we don't learn something new at work – particularly when we are newly qualified.

There are so many ways that we can learn while we work, for example:

» Practice makes perfect – a lot of us will learn more by doing than by reading. Being at work enables us to put what we know into practice and allows us to tighten up those skills that we might not have used very often.

» Experience – like everything else, the more of something we do, the better at it we get. Nursing is just the same; if we do something often we can very easily become extremely knowledgeable in that area of work. Likewise, those times when we see the conditions that we don't often deal with gives us a brilliant opportunity to learn, and the next time we see something similar we are more likely to remember what to do. The more of these experiences we have, the more we can learn from them.

» Learning from colleagues – as mentioned in *Chapter Two*, working within a team gives us many wonderful opportunities to learn from our colleagues. Wherever you work you will be surrounded by a team of people who have all come from different backgrounds and places of work. We all have unique experiences that we can share with each other, no matter how new we are to the team; we can learn a great deal from our colleagues that we wouldn't necessarily have been taught as students, and this is invaluable.

I've learned so much from my amazing nursing colleagues, and am continuing to learn more and more every shift I work. I really love working with people who have such wonderful experience and knowledge and who are happy to share this; it really makes me strive to be a better nurse. It's also brilliant to work alongside doctors, particularly those who have come from different professional backgrounds. Having discussions with them regarding how things are done in other departments allows for some great learning, and those who are training specifically for paediatrics have a really wonderful amount of knowledge about almost everything we are likely to come across, so it's amazing to learn from them. I particularly enjoy following them on their ward round because they explain things to the patients/parents using no medical jargon, meaning it's easy for me to learn and remember. I have learned to ask about anything I'm not sure of, and I don't ever think of my questions as being stupid ones; if I don't ask, how else am I going to learn? I am beginning to really enjoy passing that knowledge down to the junior nurses and students I'm working with now, and it's lovely to watch them progress. **"**

As your confidence grows

As you end your preceptorship (whenever this may be), you'll find yourself growing in confidence and truly settling into your role as a nurse. This might happen suddenly; something will click and you'll have an overwhelming feeling of self-belief, or it will happen over time and you won't even notice it. Sometimes we don't realise how much our confidence has grown, but our colleagues and patients will.

At some point, you might start to be seen as a 'senior' nurse (or as I'm often referred to, a 'senior junior'). When you get to this point you might be expected to start taking charge (if that applies to your work setting) or manage junior members of staff. Some people feel ready for this shortly after they qualify and are keen to start taking charge; you might already be interested in progressing up the bands – maybe you're ready to become a band 6? If you have this confidence that is really great!

For some people, however, this might be the last thing you're ready to do right now, but somewhere along the way there will be a time when you'll be forced to 'act up' – staff sickness can be very last minute and if you're the next most senior on shift, it's showtime! This can be extremely daunting, especially if you're not prepared; however, in some situations you have to either sink or swim. I definitely learnt this one the hard way – apologies for the length of this next personal account, but this one shift inspired almost the whole of this chapter, so it was an important experience for me.

66 *My first ever shift in charge happened around a month before my revalidation, and it was also the shift where I was caring for the most unwell patient of my career. Just one of these aspects was terrifying enough, let alone both of them falling on the same shift. I had advanced notice that I would be in charge – the band 6 went off sick the night before, and this left myself, a nurse who has been qualified for a year (but thankfully is wonderful!) who was also the only other IV giver, a healthcare assistant (who is equally wonderful) and an agency nurse who hadn't worked with us before, so we planned that I would be in charge. The night before had been a really lovely shift, so I was lulled into a false sense of security that the next night would follow suit – hahahahahaha! Who was I kidding?! I should have known that no two shifts are the same!*

When we came in for the night shift, I was told that the nurse in charge on the day shift was currently in A&E with a 12-year-old boy who was fitting. He had been given all possible medication and hadn't responded, so it was assumed that he would have to be intubated and retrieved from there. Handover ended, and within 5 minutes of stepping onto the ward I had a phone call from the consultant who was in A&E – they had stabilised the patient and were going to bring him to the ward. At the time he had a GCS of 3, so I was (understandably) terrified – I told the consultant that he wasn't safe to come to the ward with a GCS that low, but he replied that there was nowhere else for him to go, so he had to bring him down. Luckily, I'd attended a study day the week before about neurology – what to do with a fitting child; how to manage a low GCS, etc., but that didn't make me feel any better! I allocated him to myself, because I didn't think it was fair to give him to anyone else, and my fabulous second in charge already had a poorly patient.

He came to the ward accompanied by the consultant, but had a GCS of 5 on arrival (granted – this is better than the 3 he had earlier) which remained for around an hour. This was the first (and I think, only) time in my career where I was really, really scared. I didn't know what was going to happen, how I could manage it, or who I could ask for help, and I still don't know what I would have done if he had deteriorated. Thankfully, throughout the night he became more stable, and his GCS rose to 10-12 within a few hours, but he was requiring half-hourly neurological observations and therefore needed most of my time - running the ward could no longer be my priority.

This experience really knocked my confidence and it took me a long time to bounce back from it. It reinforced to me that I am not yet ready to take charge of the ward; however, it did help me realise that I am capable of managing these high dependency patients (as long as there is someone I can double-check things with). It also highlighted to me the importance of having a great team around; I don't know what I would have done without my two wonderful colleagues that night! 💬

As I mentioned previously, sometimes you either have to sink or swim; in this particular instance I sank - I ended the shift a knackered, blubbering mess. Some of my colleagues at my level or more junior would have taken it all in their stride and been absolutely fine, but not me; I just broke. That doesn't mean that I'm a bad nurse; it doesn't mean that I should never be in charge of a shift again; it just means that I'm human and I'm not ready for that level of responsibility. I think a lot of times we forget that we are allowed to be humans - nurses aren't robots - and it's a very good job we aren't. We are allowed to show our feelings and we are allowed to be scared; the trick is to not let it get us down (and try not to let our patients see - the last thing they want is a quivering wreck taking care of them). I've always known that; but it took this experience to make me really understand it.

Initially, all I could think about was how terrible that shift was, and how I never wanted to do it again, but with hindsight I started to realise how well we worked as a team that night; everything I did for my patient helped him, and within two days he had made a full recovery and was discharged home. We did everything on time, finished all of the cleaning, checked the resus trolley (something that has to be done nightly), rolled out the new observation charts that were coming into use at midnight, and we even managed to have a cup of tea together as a team. At the time this didn't feel like much, but thinking about it now, we worked amazingly that night, and I'm so proud of us!

If you've been in a similar situation and you feel like your confidence has been well and truly battered, here are some ways in which you can help build yourself up again; it might take time, but you'll get there.

» Get back on the horse – this can be hard to do and your ability to do so will depend greatly on what has happened, but the sooner you can get back to work, the better; not every day will be the same as that one, and not every situation ends the same way. I've had hard shifts where I was back the next day, and I've had hard shifts where I've had a week off afterwards, and it's always easier to get back into it the next day; time off only makes me dwell and over-think things. Try to move on from what has happened and you'll soon have your sparkle back.

» Reflect, or talk to someone – I know I keep saying this, but reflection is a brilliant way to properly help yourself understand what has happened, why it happened and how you feel about it. This can be written reflection or spoken reflection, and it doesn't always have to happen straight away; sometimes we need time to properly take it all in. I've been known to text colleagues weeks or months down the line, asking if what I did was OK and whether I could have done anything differently; it comes very out of the blue, but that's when it properly sinks in.

» Learn from it – hindsight is a wonderful thing; although it can't change what has happened, it can highlight things that could have been done differently and allows us to learn from them so that we will know what to do should we be faced with a similar situation in the future.

Further to the previous personal account, I'd like to let you know the aftermath and how it affected me as a nurse:

> 66 Around a month later, I met with my manager and 'team leader' (each member of staff is allocated a band 6 and placed in teams) to discuss my revalidation, and my annual appraisal was due at the same time. One of my reflections for revalidation was written about this incident, and my manager told me she could see that it had affected my confidence, and that she wanted to find a way to help me bounce back from it.

We talked through how I felt about being in charge and progressing to a band 6 in the future as part of my appraisal outcomes (on our ward the band 6s are the nurses in charge of the shifts and take on the coordinator role). I explained that it had completely put me off ever wanting to be in charge again, and that it made me more certain that I'm not ready to progress to a band 6 role; however, I knew that there could be times when I would have to step up and that I am prepared to do so when required. Between us we decided that the next shift I worked with my team leader (which happened to be the following Friday) I would take on the role of being the nurse in charge and work alongside her; she would show me the ropes and ensure that my experiences of being in charge were not negative ones. This shift was fine, and the experience did help me to feel more positive about being in charge now if required, but I still don't feel like I am ready to progress to a band 6 just yet. 🙥

Caring for sick patients

When you are newly qualified you're more likely to be allocated those patients who are well or 'easier' to manage; at least while you're still finding your feet and settling into your new role. As you progress, however, you may start to be given more unwell or complex patients who require more in-depth skills or knowledge than would be expected of a newly qualified nurse. When you get to the stage of taking these patients, you will find this challenge either exciting or terrifying, but try to embrace it. You will soon realise how rewarding it is to work intensively with unwell patients when they begin to recover and you can see the difference you have made.

Caring for sick patients is a great way of improving your skills and confidence, particularly when you have support from your senior colleagues. More often than not it will be an extremely positive experience; working alongside (or being supported by) a senior nurse will allow you to learn so much about managing patients with that specific condition or illness and you'll care for them brilliantly, and probably without even realising how wonderfully you're doing.

Like everything else, the more experience you have in caring for sick patients, the more confident and competent you will become at doing so; what might be a scary situation for you now will become part and parcel of the job this time next year. In order to build your confidence in caring for sick patients a mixture of knowledge and experience is required; you should know about the patient's condition, how it happens and how it affects them, the best routes of treatment and the best ways to manage it. It is in times such as these where study days and personal learning are of utmost importance, and when you are comfortable with your knowledge you can put it into practice and see the difference that you are making.

As explored in the previous chapter, there can be times when you are unexpectedly required to care for a sick patient, and if you have limited experience in this it can be really worrying. Here it is important to go back to basics; draw on your knowledge, even if you don't feel like you have much - there is always something you can do. I have attended many study days where the prospect of an acutely ill patient has been explored, and something that is always reiterated and that I've always remembered is that if you don't know what to do, go back to your initial ABCDE assessment (as recommended by the UK Resuscitation Council). By going back to the start, assessing each of these in this order and treating any problems as you go, you can ensure that you're providing your patient with the initial and most vital care that is of utmost importance. Taking it back to basics until you can find someone more senior than you to help will always be the best thing you can do, and when you know your patient's ABCDEs are all stable and you have backup and support, you will be able to help take a more in-depth look at your patient and assist in providing them with the further treatment they require. For full information on the ABCDE approach I recommend having a look at www.resus.org.uk and ensuring you are familiar with how to perform this basic assessment. You should also attend a resuscitation study day as part of your mandatory training and Trust induction, but if you feel you require more education on this, speak to your manager or practice development nurse (if applicable) and request that you be given this training.

Becoming a mentor

As a newly qualified nurse, you'll already understand the importance of having a good mentor; never forget this, because soon you will be that mentor. The first time you work alongside a student nurse can be surreal;

it might feel like only ten minutes ago that you were that student. It's a great experience to work alongside a student nurse when you're still consolidating your knowledge yourself because it can really boost your confidence and help you to realise that you do know what you're doing. Your student will in turn be able to learn a lot from you and it will help to reassure them that being a newly qualified nurse isn't as scary as it might seem.

Working alongside student nurses at this early point in your career is wonderful because it really allows you to form a unique bond, especially if they are coming towards the middle or end of their training. You'll have a lot in common, which will enable you to strike a positive relationship, and you will be able to learn new things together which will be extremely beneficial for both of you.

> **❝** When I'd been qualified for three months I was allocated to co-mentor a student nurse who was in her second year of training. I was worried that mentoring someone who was only a year and a half behind me might be difficult, but in reality I found it to be a really wonderful experience and I loved every shift that I worked with her. She was a fantastic student; already so full of knowledge and really eager to learn. In turn I found that she made me want to work harder to show her how wonderful nursing is, and I began to strive to improve my own knowledge so that I could share this with her in teaching sessions. Being able to learn new things together was lovely, but I found it so rewarding to be able to teach her practical skills and it really improved my confidence so early in my career. I'll always be so proud of her and I know that she is a truly amazing nurse. **❞**

When you become an official mentor you will get used to working with students and with time you'll discover the best ways to help them learn. This will be different for every student, so take time to get to know them, how they work and what they are comfortable with. Below is a table of Dos and Don'ts that might help you if you're allocated to mentor or work alongside a student nurse.

Dos	Don'ts
• Include your student in everything you're doing - if they have just started their training they might need to find their feet so will prefer to shadow you, but as they progress they will be able to work more independently.	• Don't just leave them to it. If your student is near the end of their training and appears competent then by all means allow them to take on their own workload, but remember that you're required to supervise them - they work under your PIN.
• You can never practise skills enough, so no matter what needs to be done for your patients, offer your student a chance to give it a try if they feel comfortable - this is a great way to learn.	• Don't push them to do anything they aren't comfortable doing. Some people prefer to watch something being done before they are willing to give it a try themselves, so allow them this time.
• ALWAYS call your student by their name; basic respect is vital and will help encourage a positive relationship between you.	• NEVER refer to them as 'the student' - I'm sure you'll remember how frustrating that can be.
• Take time to talk to them and learn what they want to take away from their placement. Have a look through their paperwork and highlight any areas that they need to improve on or that they haven't had much experience with.	• Don't just assume that they will tell you what they need to do or what they want to achieve; some people don't feel comfortable speaking up, especially on a new placement.
• Always thank them for their hard work. Asking a student to do something for you is a great way to allow them some independence, but showing them that you are grateful will help them to feel respected.	• Don't take a student for granted - having a competent student on a busy day can be invaluable, but don't treat them as an HCA; they are there to learn and they should be supernumerary.

It's important to do everything you can to make your student's training a positive experience for them, but it is equally important to remember that you're allowed to correct or challenge them, even if this might sound daunting. If you notice your student is struggling with something, take the time there and then to help them; leaving it until later might mean it gets forgotten about. If you find that they aren't working as they should, it's important to highlight this at the time; don't leave it for someone else to do. Take the student nurse aside and talk it through with them; it's about providing constructive criticism and helping them improve, not about failing them; they might not even have realised their mistake so it's likely that they will be grateful for the advice. This should be done somewhere private and you are welcome to ask a colleague to attend with you if you'd rather not be alone. If the complaint or problem is a minor one, you can work with the student to formulate an action plan for how you can move forward. If, however, the problem is a bigger one or if you find their behaviour persists, you can contact the university's link lecturer and discuss it with them. They will be able to offer advice or speak to the student themselves, but it's likely they will wish to have a further meeting with yourself and the student nurse.

Working with difficult students is very rare; most of the time you will have brilliant mentees who are extremely eager to learn. Mentoring these students is so rewarding, especially when you see them progress and grow in confidence. It's important to remember that today's students are tomorrow's nurses, and soon they could be your colleagues or the nurses caring for you or your relatives. When you're new to working with student nurses it can be difficult to know how to help them learn and how much you can expect them to know. Think back to when you were a student and the things that you found useful, and you can use or adapt these appropriately. When I was a student nurse I found one-to-one teaching with my mentor very helpful, so I try to do this with my students if we have some 'down time'. During this teaching I give them the option of what they would like to go over, if there are any skills they would like to practise or anything they are unsure about. This is a great way to help you figure out the way they learn, and it's very beneficial for them.

Sometimes, the students that we have worked with become our colleagues, and although this can be strange at first, it's really wonderful to see how well they have developed since day one. Many of my colleagues started out as students with us, and they have all become really amazing nurses who fit into the team extremely well.

TOP TIPS

★ Your preceptorship period when you first qualify will give you an important grounding in nursing and will help you get off to a great start. This time is vital because it is when you will begin to progress and if it is a positive experience it will have an amazing impact on your confidence.

★ Study days are extremely important ways to help you progress and you will find that the knowledge you receive from these days will go a long way towards helping your confidence soar.

★ Learning on the job is another extremely important way of helping your confidence grow. The more of something you do, the better you'll get at it and most people find that they learn best by 'doing'. Make the most of these valuable experiences and always find a way to learn from them.

★ As you progress you'll be expected to start caring for the sicker or more complex patients, or those requiring high dependency care. When you first start to do this it can be extremely scary, especially if you're thrown in at the deep end, but the more experience you have with this, the more confident you'll become. Having a supportive team is a great way of getting you used to caring for more unwell patients without having to feel like you're on your own, so use your team and their knowledge.

★ When you become a mentor it can be a very surreal feeling – you've gone from being the student nurse one minute to mentoring them the next. The more you work alongside students, the more you'll enjoy it, and you'll probably find that teaching someone really goes a long way in helping you to develop your confidence, as it will highlight to you just how much you really know.

WORK/LIFE BALANCE

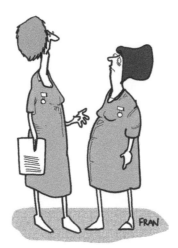

You'll have to come in over the weekend
to attend some training on managing a
healthy 'work/life' balance.

Having a good work/life balance is the key to everything in life; ensuring you make time for yourself will help you to remain more focused and positive, which in turn will mean that you're able to provide the best care that you can for your patients. This chapter will look in more depth at what a healthy work/life balance is and how you can maintain this.

Nursing is a demanding career, and if you are stressed and exhausted you are at a great risk of suffering from 'burnout'. This chapter will also explore what burnout is, how to recognise if you might be suffering from it and the best ways that you can avoid it. I will also discuss the ways in which you can support your colleagues if you think they are suffering from burnout.

Work/life balance

Whether you work full-time or part-time, long days or short days, nights, early shifts, late shifts, twilights or any combination of the above; you will spend a lot of your time at work. If you really love your job and can't think of anything else you will ever want to do (which hopefully will be most, if not all of you) it might not seem like work, but it is still extremely important that you have a good work/life balance.

Life can be a juggling act sometimes; we have so many things that we need to do and it can require some extreme planning if we want to fit it all in. You'll know from your training how difficult it can be to focus on more than just your student life, and although when you qualify you'll have less pressure to revise or write essays it can still be difficult to fit everything in. Maintaining a good work/life balance is essential in keeping you happy and healthy, and there are so many aspects to it.

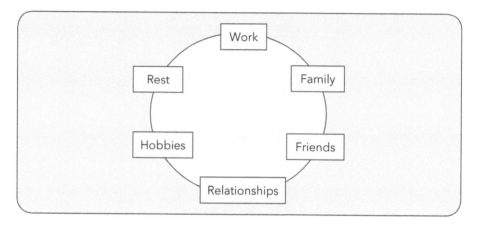

Maintaining a good work/life balance has so many benefits for yourself, your patients and your colleagues, for example:

Benefits to you	• A positive work/life balance helps you to stay happy and healthy in both mind and body. It helps to promote positive mental health, massively reduces levels of stress and helps enable your immune system to work effectively by helping you to get adequate rest. • A happier you helps to create a happier home life for yourself and your family, meaning that you're less likely to be stressed at home. • It massively boosts your job satisfaction, meaning that you're more likely to grow in skills and confidence with more ease.
Benefits to your patients	• Your patients will receive the highest possible standard of care from their focused and cheerful nurse (that's you!). • In turn they will have a more positive experience overall which can help them avoid feeling stressed and anxious while in hospital/in the community (depending on your work setting).

| Benefits to your colleagues/team | • Your positivity will have a great effect on the morale of your colleagues. This will help to improve the way your team works together and will create a wonderful working environment. |
| | • This will then act as a cycle, because the better the working environment, the less stressful it will be, meaning that you're less likely to suffer from 'burnout'. |

Nursing can be very stressful, and we face a lot of pressure both physically and emotionally. If this is all that we focus our time and energy on, we will very quickly get dragged down by it, so it is extremely important that we have a healthy work/life balance. It's really great to enjoy what you do for a living, and there is a well-known saying that goes "choose a job you love and you'll never have to work a day in your life". This is all very well and good, but even the best jobs can get on top of you if you throw everything you have at them; if all we do is work, regardless of how much we enjoy it we will quickly start to feel the consequences – stress and exhaustion will in turn lead to burnout.

What is burnout?

Burnout is generally referred to in relation to working life; people who are stressed, exhausted, overworked and unhappy in their careers are most likely to be affected. As previously stated, nursing can be a very difficult job both physically and emotionally, so people who work in settings such as these are more likely to suffer from burnout (although this doesn't mean people in other professions aren't equally at risk).

Burnout within nursing can happen to anyone at any time and can be very difficult to recover from. It is usually caused by long periods of stress, emotional or physical exhaustion or tiredness. It can be directly caused by problems at work, but can also be a mixture of work and home challenges. Burnout can creep up on you; you're busy and stressed but managing well, and then all of a sudden (usually when you stop) it hits you. Different people will experience this in many different ways, but the general symptoms of burnout include (but are not limited to):

» extreme tiredness, both physically and emotionally

» reduced sympathy and ability to connect with our patients, friends or family

» distraction and forgetfulness

» self-doubt – it can cause us to feel like we aren't good enough and can make people turn their backs on the vocation they once loved.

There are many similarities between burnout and depression, and one can lead to the other, so if you think you might be suffering from this, or if you know anyone who is, even if it's only mildly, it is extremely important that you talk about it to someone: your manager, your GP, your colleagues – anyone who can help you. Don't just keep going until you no longer can; nip it in the bud and you'll gain back control.

How to avoid burnout

Having a healthy work/life balance is one of the best ways that you can help avoid becoming 'burnt out', and it's also one of the main ways of overcoming it. Having this stable balance of work and home life allows you to enjoy both aspects more, and if you're happy at home you're likely to be happy at work. When things are going well, you'll find your self-esteem and confidence are higher, which in turn will lead to you having MORE self-esteem and MORE confidence, and the cycle will continue.

Although it is easier said than done, it is extremely important that you try to maintain this balance as best you can. Below is a list of small ways in which you can do this, and each will be expanded on as the chapter progresses.

» Have a hobby, or something to focus on outside of work.

» Leave work at work.

» You're allowed to say no.

» Take your breaks.

» Get your rest.

» Use your annual leave wisely.

» Look after yourself.

Although the above are not all concrete ways to avoid burnout, they will go a long way in helping you to stay happy and healthy both inside and outside of work.

If you are struggling with the stresses of your job it is useful to talk things through with other nurses who might be/have been in a similar position to yourself. This might be your colleagues who are experiencing the same stresses as you at work or a friend who may or may not be a nurse; although they might not understand the exact situation you're in, they will still be there for you when you need them. Alternatively, it might be someone you've never met before, such as on a social media site. I wrote about two helpful groups in *Chapter Three*: the Royal College of Nursing Students Facebook group, and the Twitter account @WeNurses. Both of these groups are extremely helpful in allowing us to express how we are feeling and ask for help/guidance from others in our profession.

> **❝** *When I'd been qualified for just over two years I found myself struggling a lot to stay positive at work. I lost my passion for nursing and couldn't seem to snap myself out of it. Instead of giving up or wallowing in it, I decided to send a tweet to @WeCYPnurses (the @WeNurses account specifically for children's nurses) asking for advice:*

> **@WeCYPnurses** help – I've recently lost my love of nursing and I'm struggling, I don't enjoy the job any more – please remind me why I started

> *The support I received from not only the people who run this group, but also the wonderful nurses who responded was incredible; I'd never met any of them, but they all sent me really encouraging messages of support, reminders of the most rewarding aspects of the job, advice about ways I can help myself reconnect with nursing and suggestions of other avenues I can try (someone who was in my position changed specialities and found a new love for her career). I was so grateful for this support and it really did help me to rekindle my love for my job, although not straight away; sometimes it's nice to talk to someone you don't know about your worries. I am still so, so grateful for the responses I received from this one tweet, and I'm sure it was those nurses who helped me find my way at that particular time.* **❞**

If your feelings are similar to mine at the time, I would definitely recommend that you talk to someone about it; whether this is someone you know or not, speaking to someone else can help you to see things from a different side and might just change your views. If you think that the speciality you're working in might be part of the problem, don't be afraid to explore some other avenues until you find your niche; they say a change is as good as a rest.

Hobbies

Part of having a healthy work/life balance means having a life outside of work. For some people, this is having a family to care for; for some it's spending time with a partner or friends and for others it is having something to do. Whatever you like to do when you're not working, it's important that you enjoy it. Having a hobby is a great way to keep a good work/life balance; it gives you something to enjoy and focus on when work is difficult. This can be any number of things – maybe you enjoy going to the gym; playing an instrument; taking a dance class; rock climbing; reading; looking at or creating art; spending time with your children or going for a coffee regularly with a friend (a retired colleague of mine used to go to a busy coffee shop weekly with her sister to 'people watch' – she said they'd spend hours doing it. It sounds like so much fun – that's a hobby I want to try!).

> " I've always enjoyed going to the theatre and since I first started working, it has been my biggest (and most expensive!) hobby. I find it a great way to escape from all of the stresses both inside and outside of work and I really, really love it. During my third winter of working I began to struggle with the pressure and stress of nursing, but at the same time discovered a truly wonderful show. I started visiting it almost weekly (they had cheap tickets for under 25s so I was making the most of the discounts before I hit the dreaded quarter century!) and it definitely became my escape, my way of de-stressing and something I really loved. Two months later that show closed, and I found that hard; my escape had disappeared, and work was still incredibly stressful. My wonderful friend and colleague suggested that I start a blog and write about the show I loved and others that I had seen. At first I was reluctant to do this as I'd never been much of a writer;

however, I set up a blog and very quickly found that I was really enjoying my new hobby. After a month I began to receive some extremely good feedback about my writing which gave me a massive confidence boost, and from then on I have found this to be my source of focus and distraction when work is difficult, and of course I still visit lots of shows too! 🙶

Finding something that you love doing outside of work will provide you with a great deal of distraction and happiness when work gets hard. Some people really love their job no matter what and will be 100% dedicated to it at all times. If this is you, that's great, but it is important to remember that work isn't everything; finding something that helps you to escape when you need it is a great way to avoid burning out.

Leaving work at work

One of the biggest causes of burnout comes from taking on too much, or putting too much of your energy into your job. Of course, while you're at work it is important that you're focused on what you're doing, but it is equally important that you're able to get away from it when you're not there. Blurring the lines between work and home can lead you to feel constantly stressed and unhappy in both aspects of your life.

Unlike other jobs, nursing is one that doesn't allow us to physically bring our work home with us; leaving the hospital premises with our patients' notes (or actual patients) is frowned upon (and illegal?!) so we don't have that stress. It does mean, however, that we can't leave work until we have actually finished everything that we are obliged to do (I know I've said earlier that it's fine to leave jobs for the next shift, but some things such as documentation need to be done ourselves).

Although we can't physically bring our work home (this largely applies to anyone below management level), we do tend to take on a lot emotionally. I'm sure we have all had our share of shifts that have had such an impact on us that we are thinking about them for days, and as much as we try to distract ourselves, it isn't always easy. I touched on this in *Chapter Four*, at the end of which you will find a list of ways to help you cope when you've been emotionally affected - have a look if you haven't already, if this is something you need advice about. The more you experience this, the better you will become at coping with it; everyone handles things differently so it might be a case of trial and error, but you'll find your way.

> 66 *A year after I qualified I attended a study day regarding a topic that most people will find emotionally difficult, and while there I met a nurse who was sharing her way of coping with the aftermath of a bad day. She told us that her drive home from work is 40 minutes, and around 20 minutes into her journey every day she drives past a specific building. When she reaches this point, she leaves her thoughts about work there and finds it very easy to continue her journey with no further worries about what has happened. I found this extremely impressive, but also a little mind-blowing; I sometimes really struggle to switch off a few days later, let alone 20 minutes after finishing my shift, but she said she has perfected this art and never has any trouble with it.* 99

If this is something that you think you could do (or even if you think you couldn't) I would definitely recommend that you give it a try; if it works for you it can be a great way to leave work at work. However, 20 minutes isn't a lot of time for you to properly reflect and come to terms with an event, especially if it is particularly difficult. If this isn't enough time for you, look back to the end of *Chapter Five* where I mentioned Sarah Millican's advice.

As important as it is to try to keep your work and home life separate, there will always be times when they overlap; a bad day at work will almost always spill over into your home life, even if it's only for a few minutes when you need a good rant to your partner/parent/friend/pet about what has happened. Likewise if you're having problems at home, whatever they may be, they will inevitably affect your work life. This can be difficult, but with great colleagues and a good support network around you, you should be able to put your focus back onto work. In some ways when it's busier at work it's better, because it can help to distract you from whatever else you have to worry about. However, if you find that you can't focus on work then it's best to talk to someone (the nurse in charge/your manager would be best, but talk to whoever you feel comfortable with) so that they can provide you with the support you need; if you lose focus you're more likely to make a mistake, so this must be avoided at all costs.

Saying no

When work is busy or there are staffing shortages, it can be tempting to take on extra shifts - whether this be bank shifts, agency shifts or time owing. Doing the odd few extra shifts is fine; but try not to overdo it. There might be times when you feel pressured into working extra, for example:

>> when your manager asks and you don't feel you can refuse

>> you put the pressure on yourself because you could do with the extra money

>> maybe you feel bad leaving your colleagues short if you don't do it and they can't find cover.

It's a very difficult situation to be in, but remember that you're allowed to say no. You might feel fine about working extra at the time, but somewhere along the line you'll get tired and that can be very detrimental to you (and if you then have to phone in sick, the ward is back to being short-staffed again). Overworking is one of the biggest causes of burnout, so although you might feel guilty for saying no, it will help you (and the ward) greatly in the long run if you take a day off to rest.

> 66 *During the first summer that I was working there were an incredible amount of bank shifts going and because I love my job and my colleagues (and because I largely had nothing else to do) I picked up a lot of extra shifts; some weeks I'd find myself doing up to five or six 12½-hour shifts. At first I had no problems with this at all; however, after a few weeks I found myself getting exhausted and emotional. I knew then that I'd been overdoing it and that I had to stop doing so many extra shifts; I now try to do two or three extra shifts a month if I can, and this seems to be a good amount.* 99

Take your breaks

We all know how busy work can be, and on some shifts it's almost impossible to get a break. However, these can be the most important part of your day; mainly because it might be your only chance to eat or drink something, or you might even get the chance to have that wee you've needed since 10 minutes into your shift! Achieving this is largely down to time management, but also the willingness to hand over some jobs to your colleagues. When I first started working I very often missed my breaks, took very short ones or went for break late because I hate leaving things for my colleagues to do. However, after around a year I began to realise that most things don't have to be done at exactly the right time; if I have obs due at 14.00 and will have a chance to go for break after this, I can do my obs (or even some medications) slightly earlier and be back from my break in time to do everything else. I've also learned that it's fine to ask my colleagues to do something for me if I really can't make time to go for a break - I do it for them! That's just another example of the importance of teamwork.

When you're on your break, you'll have the perfect opportunity to rest; eat some food, grab a cup of tea and go for that wee you still haven't had. I also try to read a book or listen to music, play a game on my phone or chat to my colleagues; anything that can take your mind off the ward for even 10 minutes will help you, particularly if you're having a stressful day. Clearing your mind will allow you to return to the ward with a fresh outlook and you'll be able to snap back into action, thinking clearly and providing wonderful care to your patients.

Around a year ago there was a poster put up around our work entitled **HALT**, the purpose of which is to remind us that we are more likely to make mistakes if we are:

Hungry

Angry

Late or

Tired.

This campaign highlights that if we are any of the above, we are not able to provide the best care for our patients, and without adequate rest we risk affecting our own physical and mental health and wellbeing. For me this acts as a very good reminder not only to take my breaks, but to use them to relax a little because of the increased risks of mistakes or poor bedside manner if I am any of the above (I've been known to get 'hangry' if I haven't at least had a cup of tea).

Take time to rest

As important as it is to ensure we take our breaks in work, it is also extremely important that we get time to relax on our days off. Juggling a busy lifestyle can mean that we often rush around from one thing to the next, without really allowing ourselves time to chill out and let our bodies and minds replenish. The importance of getting enough rest is well known, and it is widely acknowledged as one of the most important ways to help maintain good mental and physical health. Something simple such as allowing yourself a lie-in, planning nothing for your day off or allocating one evening a week (or even a whole weekend) to stay at home can go a long way towards allowing us to recover from a busy shift, and preparing us for the next one.

Resting doesn't just mean sleeping or doing nothing; it can be going for a walk, reading a book, having a bath or watching something on telly. When we take time to stop rushing around it can have a great impact on our mental health and wellbeing. Your own personal situation will determine how much rest you can reasonably allow yourself to have; for example, people with young children might not be able to rest as much as those with older children, or no children. If you have children, I take my hat off to you – having a stressful job such as nursing (whether you're newly qualified or not) alongside juggling family life is amazing – I can barely get myself ready in the morning, let alone children too. If anyone deserves a rest, it's you!

I know it's easier said than done, but you should still try to make every effort to take some time for yourself. Everyone's situation is different but listed below are some of the most common situations to be in, and advice as to how you can try to get some time for yourself:

Do you have young children or someone who depends on you?	Maybe you have someone who could babysit for you one evening so you can properly relax. 'Me time' is extremely important, and most people will be more than happy to help out. Failing that, try to put the kids to bed earlier one night; if this actually goes to plan and by some miracle they're all in bed and asleep early, the chances are that you'll then end up falling asleep on the sofa, but that's still providing you with some much-needed rest!
Do you have older/school-aged children?	There is absolutely nothing wrong with dropping the kids off at school and going back to bed, or lounging around on the sofa watching rubbish telly all day; as long as you remember to pick them up when they've finished, no one is going to mind what you've been doing!

Do you have regular commitments to someone/something?	Could you find a way to take a day off from those regular commitments, even if it is once every few weeks? No one will mind you taking time for yourself as long as there are other arrangements in place.
Do you have no children and no regular commitments?	If you accidentally sleep until 2pm on your day off, you obviously needed this sleep; if you spend all day on the sofa and don't do anything productive, you needed this time to rest. Try not to get into the habit of doing this all the time, but every once in a while is fine.

In situations such as these, it is extremely important that you **do not feel guilty** about taking time for yourself. We all need time to replenish our energy – this allows us to repair both body and mind, and will help us to recover from the stresses at work and at home. It is then easier to go back on shift with a clear view of what we can do to help provide our patients with the best care that we possibly can.

Annual leave

No matter how much you love your job, annual leave will quickly become an important source of motivation when you're working; the thought of an upcoming week or two off will get most of us through the particularly difficult shifts. It doesn't matter what you do with your annual leave days, but it is extremely important that you take them; firstly, you don't get any money back if you don't so you'll essentially be working for free (ew!), and secondly they are a great way to help you equalise your work/life balance.

> 66 *As my annual leave approaches, I always find myself counting down my days in work, regardless of how busy it's been at the time. I always try to use my annual leave to take time for myself, to get back into the hobbies I've neglected or to get away for a few days, although I largely end up doing so much that I struggle to fit it all in! No matter what I've done, I always feel refreshed when I get back to work, although the day or two leading up to going back is always when I start to reconsider whether I really need money – do I really need to work for a living?! (Unfortunately the answer is always yes; I really love food!). No matter how daunting it feels, getting back*

into the swing of working happens very quickly and during the first handover back it's like I've never been gone. **"**

TOP TIPS FOR SUCCESSFUL ANNUAL LEAVE

★ Take it - it's a sad feeling if you lose annual leave hours, even if only a day or two, so try to ensure you take what you're entitled to.

★ Enjoy it - go on holiday, stay at home and rest, redecorate your house; do whatever you want to do with it, but make sure you enjoy whatever you do. Replenish and refresh yourself and you'll soon be ready to jump back into whatever work has to offer you.

★ Try to spread it out as evenly as you can - having a week off every few months is a great way to break up the year, and helps you to avoid long periods of stress.

★ If you know a certain season is particularly busy/more stressful, try to take some leave during this time. For example, in paediatrics the winter months are usually the busiest and most heavy going (although it is becoming increasingly busy throughout the whole year), so we always try to take a week or two during November or December to allow ourselves time away from this.

★ Don't book too much bank during your annual leave - although it can be a great chance to earn a few extra pennies, it's also much-needed time to take a break, so try not to do too many extra shifts.

Look after yourself

It's worth remembering that you have to look after yourself to ensure that you are the best that you can be. Although it can be hard when working shifts, it is extremely important that you eat, drink and sleep well. In the same way as mentioned above, our busy lifestyles mean that something is usually neglected; for some people this is the chance to rest, for others it's regular meals that get missed. I know it's easier said than done (and this is where I turn into a massive hypocrite because I'm awful for this), but trying to ensure you eat and sleep well can be the most important way that you can help look after yourself.

66 *As a shift worker, I find that my biggest difficulty is estab-lishing a routine. I much prefer working night shifts; however, I still haven't properly figured out the best times to eat, how much sleep I really need between shifts or how to get myself back into 'day mode' without lying aimlessly in bed at 2am becoming annoyed because I can't sleep. I now try to organise my weeks ahead of time, planning meals and ensuring I buy snacks for when I'm working. When I'm post-nights and need to get back to being awake in the day I will set my alarm across the room so I have to get up and turn it off, or have a big drink before bed so I know I'll need to get up earlier for a wee (sorry if this is too much information, but we're all nurses here!). I'm slowly learning the best ways to tackle the irregularities of shift-working life, and I have found that my eating habits are my biggest downfall, especially on nights. I don't eat before bed, so when I wake up I'll have 'breakfast', but then I'm not hungry enough for a big meal before work so find myself snacking constantly or eating very little, but then on my days off I eat everything in the house (which I love and hate doing, in equal measures). I do find though, that as long as I plan actual meals for most days I'm fine, and I'm really making an effort to look after myself - I've no idea if it's working but I'm still alive so I must be doing something right!* 99

Supporting your colleagues through burnout

Recognising when someone is suffering from burnout is just as important as helping them through it. If you think one of your friends or colleagues might be struggling, there are many ways you can help support them, for example:

» Be a friend - listen to them and let them know that you're there when they need you. They might not want to talk at the time, but make sure they know that you're there for them when they're ready. At the time that you first talk to them about it, they might not have even realised that they're stressed, so let them come to terms with it in their own time.

» Offer them advice if you think they will be open to it, but don't make them do anything they aren't comfortable doing; don't frogmarch them to their manager or to occupational health if they aren't ready for that, as doing so will only add unnecessary stress.

>> Offer to help - this can be both inside and outside of work. Offer to babysit for them one day, or to help with that project they are working on; even taking them out for tea and cake can be a good way to help them relax and take a step back.

>> Encourage them to spread their wings (if they want to) - burnout can lead people to feel that their career isn't for them anymore, and although some stick with it and try to make it better, others will actively search for a new career or place of work. When this is a close friend or colleague, it can be tempting to try to put them off leaving because *selfishly* you'll miss working with them (I'm slowly learning the importance of not doing this); however, making someone feel guilty about leaving, whether purposely or not, can lead people to hold back from taking the next step. Encourage your friend to do what they want to do - if they're happy, so should you be; and if you don't see them at work anymore, it's all the more reason to meet up socially!

Being a source of support to your colleagues is one of the key aspects of teamwork, as highlighted in *Chapter Two*. Having good friends at work who understand what you're feeling is invaluable; even if they never need to turn to you (and vice versa), just knowing you're there can be enough to help anyone through a difficult time. Look after each other; you're all in the same boat. Surround yourself with supportive people and you're already over halfway there (sorry it's cheesy, but it's true! I don't know where I'd be without my amazing colleagues!).

TOP TIPS

★ Having a good work/life balance is one of the most important aspects of any career - remember that you're human, and you need to take time for yourself; you'll feel so much better when you do!

★ Burnout can happen to anyone at any stage in their career, and if you take on a lot of emotional stress at work this can put you at a greater risk of developing it. Having a good work/life balance can help to ward off burnout, so try to make sure you're not overdoing it.

★ Hobbies are a great way to ensure your work/life balance is equal; having something that helps you to escape when work gets busy is extremely important and will go a long way towards improving your mental wellbeing.

★ Rest is extremely important, both during work and outside of work. Taking time to put your feet up and enjoy yourself, even if just for an hour, will help you to re-energise and bounce back to being SuperNurse much more quickly. Your annual leave is a great time to do this, and being away from the stresses of work for even a week really helps you to restore an equal work/life balance.

★ If you notice that your colleague or friend might be suffering from burnout, be there for them. Be sensitive and respectful to their wishes; they might not want to talk about it, but ensure they know you're there if they need you – that will be enough.

REVALIDATION, AND EVERYTHING IN BETWEEN

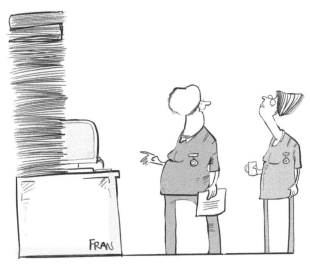

I learn something new EVERY day. Here are some of my notes from last week.

To close the book it seemed only right that there should be a chapter on revalidation. When your time to revalidate comes, you'll have been qualified for three years (at least). By now, you'll have become a wonderful and caring nurse; you might have progressed 'up the ladder' into a higher band, or even management; you might be just starting out in a new field of nursing; you might have found your niche and feel that you truly love your job; or you might still be where you started, muddling through while doing everything you can for your patients. Whichever of these you are, you should be immensely proud of yourself for what you've achieved and how far you've come. Nursing is hard, but you're the reason that your patients' stay in hospital is a positive one.

This chapter will walk you through what you need to know about revalidation, exploring each separate aspect individually and giving advice about how to get the most out of your experience. I will then explore the miscellaneous experiences that you might have at some point between graduating and revalidating. This will have less structure than the previous chapters, but will (hopefully) help remind you how far you've come and continue your love of nursing.

Revalidation

Revalidation was introduced in the UK in April 2016 by the Nursing and Midwifery Council (NMC) as a way of helping registered nurses and midwives demonstrate the safe and effective care they provide for their patients day in, day out. It encourages us to remain up to date in our practice by ensuring we take part in study days and activities that will help us continue our professional development, and encourages us to reflect on our practice by writing about our experiences and discussing them with our colleagues. Nurses must revalidate every three years, but will continue to renew our registration with the NMC yearly.

For most of us, our first impression of revalidation was that it sounded extremely daunting and lots of work - "what if I haven't completed everything I should have on time?!" Firstly, let me reassure you that revalidation isn't as scary as it sounds - when you first look at everything you need to do and compile, it seems like there is a lot to do, but most of it is done during your three years without you even realising it. I was very pleasantly surprised when it came to my time to revalidate; I met up with two colleagues who were also revalidating at the same time and we worked together to ensure that each of us had completed the requirements and compiled our evidence together. We completed it remarkably quickly, and could then spend the rest of the afternoon chatting and drinking tea - it was lovely!

If you're unsure of how to go about compiling your portfolio, have a look on the NMC website; they have templates for all of the steps involved that you simply have to download or print out and use, but outside of these templates you're free to be as creative as you want in terms of using dividers or title pages. My Trust created their own dividers that we could print off from the intranet, which highlighted exactly what we needed to include and what order it should be placed in. If you don't have this or want to try something different, there are many useful tools on the internet that you can have a look at and play around with. One tool that is particularly useful is www.FourteenFish.com which is a learning diary created for nurses and doctors to assist with revalidation and appraisals. This exists both online and as an app, and allows you to compile your achievements as you meet them, creating your portfolio once you've completed everything. It's an extremely simple and useful way to ensure that you're ready when the time comes for your final meeting, and it's really good!

So, what is involved in revalidating?

There are eight steps in total that must be completed:

>> Practice hours

>> Continuing professional development

>> Practice-related feedback

>> Written reflective accounts

>> Reflective discussion

>> Health and character declaration

>> Professional indemnity arrangement

>> Confirmation.

Each of these steps is outlined in full on the NMC website, but here I will cover what you must do for each:

Practice hours – any registered nurse or midwife (including those with a Specialist Community Public Health Nurse (SCPHN) registration) must work at least 450 hours over three years (or 900 hours if you hold a dual registration for nursing and midwifery). Although this sounds like a lot, 450 hours over three years equates to 12.5 hours every month, so it really isn't as much as it seems. If you haven't worked enough hours, you will not be able to revalidate and will have to complete an NMC-approved 'return to practice' programme before you can renew your registration. The hours that are included are any where you are relying on your skills and knowledge as a registered nurse or midwife, any time spent performing direct patient care, or any time spent managing or teaching other nurses.

Continuing professional development (CPD) – the NMC requirement for revalidation is that we must complete 35 hours of CPD across the three years, 20 of which must be participatory. This is extremely important in allowing nurses to develop in our skills and knowledge, ensuring that we are providing the most up-to-date and safe care to our patients. These CPD hours can be anything that you deem appropriate for your field of nursing, such as study days, online courses or conferences. The 20 participatory hours are any that involve input from other nurses or healthcare professionals. These can even include time spent in discussions, such as workshops. These CPD hours must be accounted for by showing evidence, such as certificates for online courses. You must also record the method of CPD, the time and date that it occurred and the aspect of the NMC Code that it best applies to. It's worth noting here that the CPD hours DON'T include mandatory training, but everything else can be used.

Practice-related feedback – you are required to submit five pieces of practice-related feedback that you have received over the three-year period. Although at first glance this might seem difficult (and random) to get hold of, they are surprisingly easy to gather – as nurses we receive feedback on our practice all the time, from cards from patients or emails praising our hard work to a 'thank you' from a patient or relative. They can include written or verbal feedback, and can be received from colleagues, patients or managers and can include your annual appraisal; as long as you can highlight how it has helped improve your practice. Chances are, over your three years you're going to be given loads of examples of this practice-related feedback, and the hardest part will be choosing which ones to submit. I got into the habit of putting all of mine into a folder when I received them, and then chose my five favourites to hand in.

> ❝ My favourite piece of feedback I've ever received came in a Christmas card from an 8-year-old, which simply said:
>
> If you weren't working on Christmas day people would die. Do you want to be a life saver or a death causer?? I hope you are very satisfied with yourself and enjoy your Christmas dinner.
>
> Aren't kids great?! This made me laugh so much and is a constant reminder of why I love being a children's nurse. ❞

Written reflective accounts – you must also include five pieces of written reflection over the last three-year period and these should be in reference to either an experience in your practice, a CPD activity and/or a piece of feedback you've received. You can follow any template you want to when writing this, and there is no requirement for how much or how little information you provide, but you must highlight if/how this experience has impacted your nursing practice and how it relates to the NMC code of conduct. The purpose of these reflective accounts is to encourage nurses to reflect on our practice; this, as highlighted on several occasions in this book, is a great way to cope with some difficult (or positive) events we have experienced and can allow us to move on from, and learn from them.

> 66 *For most people, the written reflective accounts are the most daunting aspect of revalidating. As a student, you will probably have got used to writing reflections and these are exactly the same! By now you will hopefully know what template suits you, but if you're still struggling the NMC have provided their own very straightforward template (which I used). I know it seems like a lot, but I was pleasantly surprised how simple it turned out to be!* 99

Reflective discussion – you must have a discussion about your five written reflections with another nurse who holds an NMC registration, outlining the events, how these relate to the code of conduct and how these have helped you develop or change your practice. You can decide who this registered nurse is; it can be a colleague, your manager or even someone who you don't work with often, or at all. This should be a face-to-face discussion and will help you to further reflect on the instances you have written about, providing you with an objective opinion where appropriate and providing you with an opportunity to express your feelings in person if you struggle to put these on paper. The person you choose to discuss these with will have to record their name, NMC PIN, email address, professional address and postcode on the form you will find on the NMC website. This must be done prior to completing your revalidation with your manager. I had this discussion with my manager at the same time as being completely signed off, which we have found works the best on our ward, but you can do this with whoever you wish – just ensure that you have it done in good time, so you're not rushing to fit it in before you meet with your confirmer.

Health and character declaration – this is a declaration that you are fit and well to work as a nurse or midwife, that you have no criminal convictions and are safe to practise. This is a requirement for any nurse and you must be honest and truthful; you do not need to provide any evidence to prove that you meet the requirements, just complete the declarations when finalising your revalidation. If you do not meet these requirements, you are not permitted to work as a nurse or midwife.

Professional indemnity arrangement – an indemnity agreement acts as a professional 'insurance cover'; it ensures you have financial backing available in the event of a court case or claim against you as a nurse or midwife. It is mandatory in the UK to hold a professional indemnity arrangement while you are working, so here you have to declare to the NMC that you have the appropriate cover. Most employers will provide this for you, so double-check with them that you have this. If you are self-employed then you are responsible for ensuring you have this (which you can get from most unions and some insurance companies – an internet search will show you who provides this and how to get it).

Confirmation – the final aspect of the revalidation process is the confirmation. This is where you meet with your 'confirmer' (usually your manager, but it doesn't have to be) to demonstrate that you have completed the above paperwork and are appropriately fit to revalidate. They will then 'confirm' that you have met the requirements and provide you with their NMC PIN, email address, professional address and postcode so that you can complete your revalidation.

Once you have successfully completed all of the above steps, all that's left to do is to finalise your revalidation. To do this you have to log into your NMC account to complete the revalidation application online (which opens 60 days before your renewal date) and pay your yearly fee. It is unlikely that you will have to provide the NMC with your full portfolio, but keep it somewhere safe just in case. You can store your portfolio either in paper form or electronically; it's down to your personal preference.

> 66 *For me, there is nothing better than going stationery shopping – I love it! So when it came to revalidating I took great pleasure in buying new folders, dividers and posh pens, and putting together my portfolio which I would proudly present to my manager during our meeting. You can choose whether you keep your portfolio in paper or electronic form; as long as you know where it is. Remember that your feedback is most likely to be in paper form (or card) and you'll need to print the forms for your reflective discussion and confirmation when you get signed off. You are then free to scan these onto your computer if that suits you!* 99

TOP TIPS FOR REVALIDATION

★ It's never too early to start compiling your portfolio. Things such as patient feedback (cards, emails, letters, etc.) thanking you for your care are great to include, so when you receive them, keep them safe - they will come in very handy.

★ Doing frequent written reflections won't only give you something to put towards your portfolio, they will also provide you with valuable opportunities to channel your feelings about situations and help you to learn from them.

★ Make notes of your CPD hours as you go, and save your certificates if you're given them. It's far easier to keep track of your study days as you do them, rather than trying to recap over the last three years when it comes to your revalidation.

★ Don't leave it until the last minute - your revalidation account will open 60 days before your renewal date, so book an early appointment with your manager, get yourself signed off and submit it nice and early. This way you can help yourself (and your manager) avoid the unnecessary stress of submitting last minute - if you leave it too late and your registration lapses it can mean you aren't permitted to work for up to a month until you're back on the register.

★ Fill it in with friends - chances are you will have fellow colleagues who are revalidating at the same time as you, so instead of worrying about compiling your portfolio alone, get a group of colleagues together and make it a team building exercise. If you're the only one revalidating at the time you could also contact your uni friends - you're all likely to be in the same position and if you've gone your separate ways it can be a great reason for a reunion.

Everything in between

A lot happens between the time you graduate and the time you first revalidate; those three years will go by very quickly, and it's only when you stop and look back on everything you've achieved that you'll realise how far you've come and how amazingly you've done.

So far, this book has covered the vast majority of the experiences you'll generally have while working, and although not everything will be applicable to every branch, speciality, place of work or individual person, aspects of it are relevant to almost every nurse working in every sector. Some aspects of nursing, however, have gone undocumented, partly because of my own inexperience of them, and partly because they just don't fit under any particular topic. Below you'll find some of these more miscellaneous experiences that can happen to you throughout your years of nursing. These also don't just apply to your first three years, but throughout your career as a whole; they might have already happened, they might be about to happen, or they might never happen. Each of us is different in the way we nurse, in our thoughts and in our opinions, but these are some things that I can say have stood out for me in my career so far.

Nursing changes you

There is no denying that your role as a nurse will have some impact on you as a person; there are so many ways in which it can change you for the better. Whether this is your personality, your knowledge of certain topics or your general views, beliefs or opinions, no one can say that they have not been in some way affected by their nursing career.

At some point along the way you will grow an enormous backbone; whether you start out as a shy mouse or an already ferocious lion, nursing can put you into situations that will require you to speak up, either for yourself, your colleagues, or most frequently, your patients. The more you have to do this, the more confident you'll become. When you start out you might find it difficult to speak up when you disagree with a doctor, a patient or a relative, but in times when you really feel that your patient will suffer, you'll be surprised at how well you can do this.

> 66 *When I started work, one of my colleagues called me 'Mary Poppins' because (she said) I am always calm and cheerful, and I love working with children. After I'd been qualified for around 2½ years I worked with that colleague again for the first time in a while, and she asked: 'What happened to the shy and quiet newly qualified nurse you were?! You used to be Mary Poppins, but now you're more like the Wicked Witch of the West!'. At first I was slightly offended, but she explained that she simply meant I am no longer afraid to speak up and voice my opinion if*

it's something I really care about. I now realise exactly what she means; for years I was so shy I wouldn't say boo to a goose, but now I am quite comfortable with speaking up when I feel that something isn't right. This might make me seem like a Wicked Witch, but if I know that I am helping my patients by doing this, then I'm happy! **""**

Nursing can also harden you to certain things; when you experience the range of emotions that are prevailing within your job you might find yourself becoming tougher, which can spill over into your personal life. This isn't necessarily a bad thing, but be careful not to let yourself become too cold; if you let it affect you too much you might risk becoming unfeeling or unsympathetic. Empathy is a critical component of providing compassionate care; it will be your best friend, so don't lose it.

You'll make lifelong friends

It's very rare that you'll ever work within a team of people that you don't form friendships with; even if there are only one or two. The beauty of having friends at work is that they can understand exactly what you're going through in tough times, and together you can celebrate the great times - you're all in it together. A lot of this was covered in *Chapter Two* with regard to teamwork, so I won't go over it too much here, but I think it's extremely important to remember that your colleagues will be your rocks on so many occasions, and if you're lucky enough to be part of a really good team, cherish them.

Both as a student and as a qualified nurse I have made good friends with those I have worked with. Nurses by nature are so kind and supportive, meaning that no matter where you go you'll be welcomed as an important part of your new team. I am blessed to work with the most amazing group of nurses I've ever met, and every shift I work with them makes me more and more grateful. There is nothing more special than being part of a team like mine; a bad shift is made that little bit better by the colleagues we've been working with, and good shifts are celebrated that bit more because of those we've enjoyed them with. Cherish your colleagues, and welcome new members to your team (this includes members of the multidisciplinary team too, not just nurses) and you'll be part of a team you can really be proud of!

One of the best things about having nurse friends is that you all have the same sense of humour; there are some things that I would never discuss with my non-nursing friends, a) because they probably wouldn't really understand what I am nattering on about, b) because they would think I have a twisted sense of humour and c) I would definitely put them off their dinner. Having nurse friends means that we can have all of these weird and wonderful discussions and none of us thinks they are odd.

> 66 Just after I'd started university I was sitting at the dinner table with my family and discussing the things I'd been learning about with my parents (who are both also nurses). We were in the middle of a full-on discussion about UTIs when we turned to look at my brother, whose face showed that he clearly didn't have a clue what we were talking about – it's easy to forget that other people don't really understand this kind of conversation, and that talking about urine at the dinner table is actually quite gross. 99

You'll find your niche

As a student nurse your variety of placements will give you the opportunity to try to figure out where exactly you want to work. For some people, this is enough time to truly find their niche, but some people still need more time; there might be so many specialities that you enjoyed that you still don't really know which path you want to follow. This is absolutely fine, and just because you've been employed somewhere doesn't mean you're stuck there; you're allowed to move around until you find where you truly love working. It's better to try lots of places of work before you really settle in, than to stay somewhere because you feel like you should.

There are so many factors that affect your decision about moving somewhere new or staying put, such as:

» the type of job – if you're working in a speciality that you have no interest in, it can be harder to want to remain there

» your lifestyle – if where you're working suits your lifestyle, for example if the hours suit you for childcare, then you're more likely to stay there

>> your team - working with a great team can help you to love your job, whatever the field you're working in

>> the geographical location - although it might not be your first choice of speciality, working closer to home might be your biggest priority and the reason that you stay/move somewhere.

> *As a student nurse there was only one place that I wanted to work when I qualified; a very well-known children's hospital in London. I applied to work there, but I didn't get a job working in the speciality that I wanted so decided to stick with the first job I'd been offered; a rotation within a district general hospital that would last for 18 months. My original plan was that I would do this rotation to give me a good grounding in three different areas of work, and then I would be able to reapply to work in the hospital that I'd had my heart set on. This plan changed very quickly when I settled into the job that I am doing now, and I no longer have any interest in specialising in any particular aspect of nursing; I love working on a general ward as I get to build up skills in so many different areas. Although it wasn't in my original plan, I am so happy that everything worked out the way that it did, as I have well and truly found my niche.* >>

No matter how long it takes you, when you find your niche you will see a completely different side to nursing, and you will love it all over again!

Sometimes you'll grow an unfathomable confidence

I don't know whether this one is down to nursing or human nature, but there will be some shifts you work that will instil in you some type of amazing confidence. You'll feel like SuperNurse; your patient care will be second to none, you'll do absolutely everything that is required of you (and more), and you'll really feel amazing. When this does happen it's the best feeling ever (even if it does only last for one shift) and it goes a long way towards building up your confidence.

> *Throughout my whole career I've always lacked confidence in myself and my work - more often than not I finish a shift convinced that I haven't been good enough; I know deep down that this isn't true, but the worry is there. However, I have*

occasional shifts where I suddenly feel invincible; I feel like I can do anything, help anyone and make a real difference to my patients, their families and my colleagues. I have one of these shifts on average around once a month, which I know isn't very often but I never see them coming, so when they do happen I suddenly get an overwhelmingly positive feeling of confidence. I know that I provide the best care I possibly can on every shift I work, but shifts such as these really help me to realise that I am a good nurse. **"**

Whenever you have a shift like this, it might be worth reflecting on it; think about what you did that was amazing, what you might have been doing that made this shift different to others you've had, and how you can move forward in making sure these types of shifts become more frequent. By doing so, you can try to help yourself realise that you can be this 'SuperNurse' much more frequently.

There are many reasons why you might have shifts like this:

» Your mood – if you're feeling positive about work then this will be reflected in the way you nurse.

» Your colleagues – if you're working with people who you work very well alongside, this can be a massive influence. In another way, if you're working with more junior colleagues, this can impact your confidence in a positive way; when you're seen as 'senior' it can help you to feel more self-assured in your work and your decisions.

» Your patients, and their conditions – if you're looking after a patient who you know, or who has a condition that you're knowledgeable about or confident in caring for, then you're automatically going to feel great about caring for them.

Focus on your patients, and do all that you can to give them the best care that you possibly can, and you're already a SuperNurse!

You'll still get scared, but you'll learn from these moments

This is almost the opposite of the above point, but it is something else that you will experience along the way. As I have established in previous chapters, the longer you're qualified, the more confident you'll become in your nursing role. However, there will still be shifts that will test you and patients who will suddenly take a turn for the worse and scare you. As experienced as you might be, you will still have moments where you really don't know what to do (our patients are good at keeping us on our toes, aren't they?!). In these moments it is important to remember to try to keep a calm and logical head on your shoulders; don't panic, don't flap, just get help and do everything you can for your patient – they are your number one priority at all times.

> 66 As I have previously mentioned, the winter months are the busiest in children's nursing, and it is during this time that we see mostly patients with respiratory illnesses. Most of these children present with the same or similar symptoms, so usually they are all managed in very similar ways. We get very used to managing these patients, and by January are so used to doing this that we can almost do it in our sleep. Patients are tricky though, aren't they? Sometimes, we are doing everything that would normally help any other patient, but there is one who doesn't play by the rules and despite our best efforts, they go downhill. In my mind, there are several different strategies that can be tried when certain things happen, and nine times out of ten at least one of these will work. When they don't, however, and we run out of options, it can get scary very quickly and I just don't know what to do. This is the most horrible feeling; as a nurse all we want to do is help our patients get better and when this doesn't work it can be terrifying. 99

Interestingly, in the same way as you will have moments of invincibility, you will have similar moments of worry that come out of the blue and might knock your confidence; something that you've been doing with ease on previous shifts might become very difficult on one random shift (this again might be more to do with human nature than nursing, and might not happen to everyone). If you find yourself having one of these shifts, just do all that you can to help your patient; get them reviewed by a senior nurse and a doctor and provide them with the most appropriate treatment that you can. As long as you haven't done anything that will bring your patient to harm, and you have done the best you can, that's all that you can do.

You'll learn something new every day

Nursing is one of those amazing professions that is always changing; research is constantly being done that will show us ways to provide better care for our patients, highlight symptoms earlier than might have been the case, and introduce more improved treatments for their conditions.

Nursing has changed so much just in the three years that I've been qualified, and there is always something new that we can learn. Every day you're at work you'll be learning, and that's so exciting! As the evidence changes, so must our clinical practice; keeping an open mind about the care you're providing is the only way to ensure you're being the best nurse you can be. Don't be afraid to move with the times – that's the only way development will happen.

As previously noted, attending study days is a great way to stay on top of the frequent changes and updates in practice, but that's only the first step; knowing about the developments is great, but you have to pass these on to your colleagues and use them in your practice in order to really make a difference.

Study days aren't the only way to develop your knowledge, however. Talking to your colleagues about things that they have learned is also a great way to enhance your practice. Doctors often have very extensive teaching sessions so that they are kept up to date with the latest research and developments, so if a doctor recommends that you try something new, don't dismiss it – as long as you can't find any reason that it wouldn't work (for example any contraindications should be addressed and reviewed), then give it a try. It is in this way that we can really learn more about the conditions our patients have, and the ways in which we can help treat them and really make a difference to our patients' lives.

You might also learn something that might change your perceptions or opinions on some topics. In your nursing role you're going to meet people and experience things that might influence you to change a long-held opinion you once had. There is absolutely nothing wrong with this; it's better to let this happen than to get stuck in your ways. Nursing allows us to get to know people from loads of different backgrounds, who have had a wide variety of experiences; whether this is our colleagues, our patients or their relatives. Learning about them, their lives and their opinions or beliefs can influence our own, and this can be a wonderful thing to experience.

This can refer to any number of examples, from something small such as an opinion about how something should be done, to something more significant such as a belief you once held. This can be difficult when you first become aware of it, particularly if your perception has been changed regarding something that you once really fought for. It's OK to be open-minded and realise that your point of view has changed; it just shows that you are growing as a nurse and as a person.

Nursing has a huge impact on your life

No matter how long you've been nursing for, from the day you started you'll have already felt the impact on your life. The way this happens will be different for all of us, but you'll definitely feel yourself changing because of it. Nursing will shape you as a person, it will help you to realise the important things in life and it will bring you so much joy when you see the impact you're making on your patients. Yes, nursing is hard, and it probably isn't going to get any easier, but when you think about all of the lives you've already changed, and the lives you've yet to change, you'll remember the wonderful impact you're making.

Nursing really is wonderful, and nurses really are wonderful! Keep going, have faith in yourself and always remember that you are SuperNurse!

ACKNOWLEDGEMENTS

There are so many people I need to thank for their endless support, not just while writing this book but throughout everything. I will try not to make this sound too much like a BAFTA acceptance speech (but it is the closest I'll ever come to winning a BAFTA so I might as well milk it!).

Firstly, to my amazing work family; you're such a wonderful source of support and guidance, and I would not have survived this far without you - we are definitely the Dream Team! A particular thank you to my wonderful friends; the Awesomes (Amy, Jade, Claire and Emma), my Breakfast Buddies (Becki, Marie, Lisa and Lisa) and Magnificent Maggie; the nurse in charge on my first ever day at work who blew me away with her madness and hilarity! Your support and friendship have meant so much; you are all amazing and you make me strive to become a better nurse.

Thanks to Dee, my lovely housemate who has had to put up with me wittering on over the last six months. Thanks for not getting fed up with my constant reading out loud and asking "Is this funny?", and "does this make sense?!"

So many people have helped me in terms of content, from proofreading parts to giving advice regarding how things happen and how you felt at the start; a special thanks to Laura, Amy and Lisa for your help and input with this.

My parents are both nurses, and although they tried to put me off nursing (by making sure I knew the reality of the job), they've always supported me in my training and career, so thanks Mum and Dad.

Thank you to the team at @WeNurses and the RCN Students Facebook page for your guidance and support throughout my writing this. I've had a lot of input from student nurses that I've connected with on social media; a massive thanks to you all for your contributions, particularly Francesca, Marie, Poppy, Lauren, Rachel, Naomi and Jasmine.

A big thanks to Peter and the team at Lantern for giving me the opportunity to share my experiences with you all - I've loved writing this book so much!

A MASSIVE thank you must go to Marie – your support and encouragement to start writing really opened up so many doors for me and you helped me to realise that I'm actually not half bad at it. I never would have thought to start blogging if it wasn't for you, and I'm so, so grateful!

The final thank you goes to those of you who are reading this. I hope that this book will help you through the good and bad days, and I hope you enjoy reading it as much as I've enjoyed writing it.